T0354643

SEX AFTER SEVENTY: IT GETS BETTER

The Detailed Sex Guide for Mature-Thinking Adults and for Seniors

JAMES A. GRANT

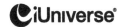

SEX AFTER SEVENTY: IT GETS BETTER
THE DETAILED SEX GUIDE FOR MATURE-
THINKING ADULTS AND FOR SENIORS

iUniverse books may be ordered through booksellers or by contacting:

iUniverse
1663 Liberty Drive
Bloomington, IN 47403
www.iuniverse.com
1-800-Authors (1-800-288-4677)

ISBN: 978-1-5320-4580-6 (sc)
ISBN: 978-1-5320-4581-3 (hc)
ISBN: 978-1-5320-4584-4 (e)

Library of Congress Control Number: 2018904564

Print information available on the last page.

iUniverse rev. date: 09/07/2018

CONTENTS

WARNING:
IF YOU HAVE AN IMMATURE ATTITUDE TOWARD SEX, DON'T
READ THIS BOOK. YOU WON'T UNDERSTAND IT.

AN OVERVIEW AND INTRODUCTION

"SEX IS THE MOST POWERFUL BIOLOGICAL AND EMOTIONAL FORCE IN OUR LIVES AND MOST OF US KNOW VERY LITTLE ABOUT IT."

NOTE: Please pay particular attention to "earthquake machine" in Chapter IV. It's not what you would expect.

One of my favorite statements is that people with small minds like to gossip and talk about other people. People with medium sized minds like to talk more about events, and that people with larger minds like to talk more about ideas. The idea in this book is this: SEX IS THE MOST POWERFUL BIOLOGICAL AND EMOTIONAL FORCE IN OUR LIVES AND MOST OF US ACTUALLY KNOW VERY LITTLE ABOUT IT. In one way or another it influences nearly ALL of our decisions. It can influence where we choose to go to school, where we choose to live, where we work, who we will share our life with, what our financial future will be and virtually any other important life decision. Sex is for procreation, for pure pleasure, and for the most sacred bonding between partners. On the other hand, we have been trained by the pervasive use of sex in our society to trivialize its true importance, and despite all of the innuendo and superficial exposure, we really know very little about the facts of our sexuality and how to use it in a healthy way. Sex shapes our personalities and dictates our future in every way. There is a sexual component to all human relationships and even the most casual interactions. Despite that, serious sexual discussions rarely occur that actually transfer vital and specific enough information to allow us a healthy outlook and understanding of our true selves and how we relate to others.

One might think that as much as I make of sex in this book, that I think sex is the most important thing in the world. Not at all, but what I do think is that we have not understood the incredibly strong position that sex plays in our moods, our reasoning, our decisions and our relationships, thereby directing our lives in ways that we aren't consciously aware of. We could list the usual things such as world peace, world hunger, absence of diseases, and numerous other things that are more important than sex, but the solutions to all of those are really more academic than something any of us as individuals can really do substantially about fixing. We can do something about the quality of our personal sex lives. Making more harmonious personal relationships one by one on a grander scale then translate into a more harmonious world.

My initial interest in writing this book was to address the elephant in the room that nobody would talk about. I had long observed an extreme unsettledness in menopausal couples, but then realized that in a long life of observation and some unsettledness of my own, that younger couples really needed someone of longer experience and good intent to guide them in specific techniques and hard earned life lessons. In other words I thought it was time for someone to candidly talk to them about those extremely delicate things that make us all instinctively blush so that they don't waste many years either unfulfilled or only mildly aware of their own sexual potential. The younger crowd might not be fully ready for all of the concepts in this book such as menopause or infirmity, but they do need to know what to expect so that when it hits them they won't be overwhelmed. They will also definitely benefit from the techniques passed on to them that only years of experience and some study can give them. This book is written by a Christian for Christians and everyone else. However, you will notice as you read on that I don't take the dogma that is commonly taught from pulpits as unquestionable truth by a few people who would like you to believe that their own interpretations or their particular brand of religion is the infallible truth. Call me a renegade if you wish, but I prefer to do my own thinking rather than have my thinking dictated to me. I encourage you to do the same.

WHAT SHOULD YOU BELIEVE AND WHY?

Throughout this book, I use bits and pieces of programs, seminars, videos, individual statistics, magazine articles, and life experiences, etc., some of which are anecdotal, along with highly documented scientific studies by qualified experts because I don't intend this to be a scholarly work, but a general help source. I believe that we benefit from overall knowledge which is the combination of anecdotal knowledge, and personal experiential knowledge, as well as from scientific studies. I have seen instances where all types of sources are correct and instances where all types of sources are incorrect. Use your own judgement as to what you decide to believe and what you don't. What I write in this book is an informed and studied opinion of an observant person who has lived a long time, and if it has the ring of truth to it, use it to make your sex life more skilled and increase your sexual contentment. On the other hand, if you don't see validity in my studied points of view and conclusions, be content with the common degree of sex skill that you have now and don't do anything to improve it. Although I cite sources and studies which have gratefully become a part my knowledge, I am not interested in documenting this book as a scientific work because it is not. For those who believe that everything is provable and documentable, I wish to say "Please sell me two pounds of love for the market rate". There is no quantifiable way to measure love and no measurable way to price an unmeasurable concept that we all know exists, but can't prove. Anything regarding emotions is difficult or impossible to actually quantify or prove, but we know it when we see it.

THE "YUCK" SYNDROME AND THE SOLUTION

There is a classic joke about walking in on your parents "doing it" and it always elicits a shocked "EEEWWWWW" kneejerk disgust response to think of two overweight, wrinkled, and seemingly uninteresting people actually going at "IT". That is what we are supposed to think, isn't it? That is only what you see on the surface. It is likely that you may be uninformed about the vast body of recent knowledge, skills, and tools that some of those older people have added to the knowledge they had already gained through many years of experience. Today, more and more skilled people know how to arouse and completely satisfy the same mate for decades after the exuberance of youth has disappeared. That's no small task because sex with the same person, even if you dearly love them, gets boring. That goes for the young as well as older people. I know that is something that is hard to admit, but it's true. If you are a thirty something, you might not have experienced that yet, but you will. If you are post-menopausal, you know exactly what I mean. You actually have to know something about the very DIFFERENT KINDS

OF ORGASMS and how to skillfully coax them to a level just barely below climax and bounce along the edge for long periods before choosing exactly when to bring down the curtain of one or even several deeply satisfying orgasms. That takes skill and finesse and even some equipment. If you haven't experienced all of the different types of orgasms you still have room to learn more. That alone can stretch the boredom cycle out to a longer interval so that sex becomes less predictable. The skill is learning how to attain orgasms at will and without effort. You can learn to experience all different types of high level orgasms and also learn to control them much easier than you did when all you had was youthful enthusiasm and overabundance of raging hormones, but very little real skill. After reading this book and applying what you read, you will be able to do just that. You will definitely learn some things you don't already know and your sex skills will improve no matter what your age is.

GOOD SEX IS A LEARNED SKILL

Despite what we all would like to believe, GOOD SEX IS A LEARNED SKILL. Good sex doesn't come naturally to most people without some specific study and practice. WE ARE NOT BORN WITH THE SKILL TO HAVE REALLY GOOD SEX. When you are that ultra horny teenager overflowing with hormones, it isn't necessary to have so much skill to have an orgasm, but that won't always be the case. Sex becomes a somewhat more deliberate action as one ages. Skill is needed to offset the loss of an overabundance of the exploding hormones of youth and to become consistent at satisfying your mate effortlessly. The real skill is in knowing exactly how to time every motion and exactly what touch to use to have complete control over the entire sexual experience. All steps are important and include creating the mood, becoming lost in the moment and oblivious to all surroundings, building the sexual tension, and then literally coasting to the climax of only one orgasm if that is all you desire, or to multiple orgasms of varying kinds if that is what you desire. The second secret is to learn to do it effortlessly so that the experience is fun and fulfilling and isn't an ordeal. In order to accomplish that, you will probably have to learn much more about your own body and more about your mate's body than you presently know.

BODY LANGUAGE AND MICRO BODY LANGUAGE

You can become so aware of your own and your mate's body language AND micro body language that your sexual awareness and responsiveness is greatly magnified. You are probably at least somewhat familiar with body language, but in sex, it is the micro body language that you must also learn to identify and use to be effective. Micro body language is discussed in more detail later in the book. What a difference it is to have sex with a partner that projects and receives all of the subtle signals we all use to communicate sexually! It is much easier to learn from someone who has been there and done that rather than learning the slow and difficult way by wasting years of good sexual energy and consuming good relationships. Have you ever seen that information offered anywhere? I haven't, and that's another reason I am writing this book. It is for younger adults as well as postmenopausal adults. This book will help you tune your sexual transmitter and receiver to function more effectively. As an important side benefit, the knowledge will reach outside the sexual realm to make you a more effective communicator in general relationships.

SUBSTITUTION AND DIVERTING ATTENTION
DOESN'T WORK TO SOLVE THE REAL PROBLEM

Humans are affected by sexual tension from before puberty onward. That tension manifests itself even more pronounced as menopause approaches. Lack of focus and concentration is one common symptom for younger people, and almost all postmenopausal women are perpetually frustrated and don't have a clue why they are always in such a condition. Many suffer from chronic insomnia that can ultimately affect their health. For many years I have observed them in their nervous quest for a satisfaction and fulfillment and that included my own mother. I have seen people substitute anything from religious fanaticism, gardening, a cat or dog, bridge clubs, social butterflying, over-involvement with the minutia of grandchildren's lives, civic activities, and dozens more things that divert their attention from the real problem of an unfulfilled or ignored sex life. These activities are just fine in their proper amount and priority, but when they are used as a substitute for a fulfilling sex life, trouble is brewing. This typically starts when their husbands lose the overrated ability to have instant and hard erections causing their husbands lose their male confidence and lose interest in satisfying the sexual needs of their mates. It could also start with their husbands developing a wandering eye caused by the wife's complacency or disinterest.

The husband and the wife must become aware of the vital role of the production and regular release of hormones and pheromones that is biologically necessary to all persons' sexual wellbeing and biological balance as long as we still breathe. When the husband puts too much time into playing golf, hunting and fishing, over indulgence with grandchildren, or fanatically chasing a hobby, you can bet that his mate will start doing the same and their sex lives will seriously diminish rather than build the expert level of sexual fulfillment that will ensure a healthy biology in advanced age. The results of ignoring this vital component of life ranges from a boring and unfulfilling stalemate relationship to divorce in many extreme cases.

YOUTH DOESN'T KNOW IT ALL

The next paragraphs are mostly for young people, but you old farts are welcome to read them because I guarantee some of it will strike a chord.

Most of us think we know quite a bit at age 35. I thought that I did. At age 50 I realized how little I really knew when I was 35. At age 70, I realize that I had just only awakened at the advanced age of 50 and have learned at least as much AFTER age 50 than I did before age 50. That goes for everything---including sex. In other words, because of more years of archived experiences and cross referencing the years of experiences with an analytical and curious mind, I believe that my life knowledge has doubled in just 20 more years. I fully expect that trend to continue at an ever increasing rate throughout life, but it doesn't just happen without some sort of directed effort. I am nothing special, and anyone can do the same with a little curiosity and a sense of purpose.

SEX IS SO NATURAL THAT YOU REALLY DON'T NEED ANY INSTRUCTION, ISN'T IT?

Getting pregnant is natural. Good sex isn't.

Just think about it logically for a moment. Who actually

TAUGHT you how to have sex? Was it your father, your mother, a friend, a curious cousin, or did you actually think that your instinct was all you needed to use with trial and error to stumble and blunder your way to expert level? We all talked about it and thought about it incessantly, but none of us knew much more than where to put what, but not how to really be effective. We all knew that having an orgasm was as easy as falling down and we just trusted instinct to make wonderful things happen. Because it was so easy, we thought that we just do the same thing over and over again. Since small successes continued to be so easy, we just assumed that we were super stud, or super diva. The clitoris was sticking out like a face on Mount Rushmore and so our sex life centered upon our wonderful discovery and we stopped looking for the really hidden more sophisticated sexual treasures. What most of us didn't realize was that were settling for topping our sexual abilities at a low level because it was easy to let our ego lull us into thinking we were better than we really were. We actually stunted ourselves because we had found something that worked and just stopped looking to see if there was still more to learn. We likely never really put ourselves in the roll of a student and we didn't actively go after the information that would make us more highly skilled. We just grabbed bits and pieces as we could with no real conscious course of learning. It might have been our fault if there was really a place we could easily access useful information in one place, but there wasn't. The information was sketchy to non-existent, scattered all over, and much of what I will be addressing in this book wasn't widely known. As wonderful as Miss Clitoris was, we missed out on all of the best parts because we stopped actively trying to learn more about her friends. How could we have known that the rest and the best secrets were still hiding under the surface and out of sight, protected from the hordes of casual and ignorant who would defile them without the proper respect and finesse!

IF YOU SKIP READ THIS BOOK YOU WILL MISS A LOT

I have woven some of the specific physical and mental techniques all throughout the book purposefully repeated and scattered so that their discovery will be mixed with other relationship information. I have purposely repeated several key bits of information throughout the book, each time adding a little more information with it. I believe the repetition will help in the learning process and presenting a given point repeatedly, but slightly differently also aids in retention. I want you to have to type in internet searches when you run into words you are not familiar with so you can ground your new knowledge with your own efforts. If you don't read the book in its entirety, you will miss many key words and important bits of information. My hope is that it will encourage those people who just want to take shortcuts to examine the whole picture and understand that it is the entire relationship that sets the stage for success. This entire book can be read in under 4 hours which is just a typical evening of television. It isn't a large commitment of time, but the rewards are great if you will commit just that amount of time to understanding yourself and your mate. Then, the goal is to work out the details of physical and psychological parts of sexuality together which is tailored for your own individual sex lives based on where you see your own personal areas of misinformation, disinformation or lack of information. We have all been inadvertently influenced by misinformation and purposefully influenced by disinformation, and restricted through lack of information.

HORMONES AND PHEROMONES ARE POWERFUL

Ladies, I hate to pop your party balloon, but it isn't any big achievement to be able to get a hormone dominated 18 year old lad stimulated to an erection. His organ will rise like baked bread many times a day (and night) whether you personally are around or not. Just about any female within the radius of a football field makes it happen just by being there. Your oozing pheromones that you had absolutely zero control over misting around you continually, put that 18 year old lad under your spell. The lad didn't even know what hit him. That has to be a huge power trip for young ladies, but that power diminishes with time as your shining physical beauty and your pheromone and hormone production levels come down out of the stratosphere. When that inevitably happens, you will need some other skills to augment your feminine wiles. There might be a time when you are competing with ladies 20 or more years younger than you are who are still profusely oozing all those powerful natural chemical potions around your husband while your own magic potions are on the wane. Is that really a good time for you to be lax in maximizing your attractiveness? No, it is not! As the boredom sets in and you pay less and less attention to making yourself desirable to your mate, it is precisely NOW that making yourself the most interesting sexual being you can in every way is the most important thing you can do. Those hormones are nuclear bombs and you'll need to know more about what is happening in your body and your mate's body. Now is the time to "be all you can be". Add to that, the other woman, just about ANY other woman, saying just the right thing to stroke the faltering ego of your mate can turn even the most well intentioned heads. Another woman batting her eyelashes with just the right smile is like a live worm dangling an inch in front of a hungry trout. You can no longer just lay there passively and be a mildly interested bed partner wearing your jeweled crown while you passively and unpassionately spread your motionless legs if you want a lifetime of love and full devotion from your mate. This wandering eye syndrome happens at any age, and it can happen with both men and women, so the dispassionate attitude goes both ways.

SEX IS A PHILOSOPHY

This next few paragraphs might seem irrelevant at first, but actually they are dead on target.

I was a karate instructor and taught classes to earn college money as a young college student. The greatest failing of many new students was that they wanted to learn how to become a "bad ass" before they learned the most important defensive skill. That most important skill is how to actively avoid verbal conflicts that lead to physical violence.

With the correct philosophy you can, and should, avoid physical conflicts by deflecting verbal violence that can escalate to physical violence. Your controlled physical skills should be used strictly for defensive purposes and are to be used only when absolutely necessary. One of my biggest challenges as an instructor was making students realize that karate and other martial arts aren't about becoming a "bad ass". (Ego has to be put aside in favor of preventing harm to come to anyone, including the aggressor). The sensei (teacher) was responsible for teaching attitudes and techniques to control deadly learned skills through an inner peace and confidence of really knowing that you could deflect any attacker with honed skills whether the attacker was armed or not. Most new students had a hard time assimilating the philosophy that by learning how to defend yourself, you learn to become confidently passive. You learn how to avoid conflicts and deflect violence by having the verbal and physical skills to nullify the aggression of others, both with words and physical skills. Note that I also included verbal violence which is the first step to a deteriorating incident headed for combat, or just as aptly, to a combative attitude in a relationship. It is a philosophy that is applicable to all relationships. The philosophy you have toward sex will determine your success and skill level as a sexual partner and will have a bearing on your ability to relate to others on a general level. This isn't just some kind of mystical crap. THE CONFIDENCE YOU GAIN FROM REALLY BEING IN FULL CONTROL OF YOUR SEXUALITY MAKES YOUR MOVEMENTS DRASTICALLY MORE EFFECTIVE AND EFFORTLESS. By using the philosophy that you wish to avoid conflict in your relationship and to raise your skills so that you can control your own actions and the actions and reactions of your partner with correctly intentioned skill, you become the master of your own sex life. Simply put, when you really know what you are doing, you will become an expert and you will be in control.

LEARN TO CONTROL YOUR SEXUALITY

You can become so skilled by applying what is in this book that you will have complete control of your sexuality. It becomes a philosophy of knowing that you have the correct attitude and the skill of transmitting and receiving the necessary sexual signals to maintain harmony, cooperation, and enthusiasm from your mate. It should become your philosophy to give all you can to your mate. All that you give will be returned in greater measure to you. You have read and heard about this philosophy before---"do unto others---"? You know the rest.

This book is definitely about very specific sexual knowledge and techniques that are described in such a detailed way that it can be really useful and not just generalized innuendos that are in many "how to" books already in print. A couple of the chapters are pretty graphic, but I don't apologize for them because I am only reporting what is reality and you will need the details in order for the information to be effective. You can attain new knowledge and learn the skills that most people don't have so that you are in REAL control of your sex life if you are willing to act as a student and open your mind to learning new skills. This book will first give the vital philosophy that sets the stage for a deep and respectful relationship including the reverence for your own body as well as the body of your mate. Then, and only then, will you be ready to implement the physical techniques to their fullest potential of both partners in a relationship.

My goal is for you and your mate to recognize the philosophy that makes all close relationships work if you have temporarily let the vitality slip away. Then use that philosophy to raise your level of knowledge and skills and become fully in control of your sexual ability. Of course it is better to learn it young so that you won't waste years of your life, but because you have fewer years to practice it, apply it if you are post-menopausal so that your golden years will really be golden.

IT'S TIME TO LEARN SOME OF THE NEW BIOLOGICAL INFORMATION

Much specific and remarkable new knowledge about human sexuality is available now that wasn't available until fairly recently. Unfortunately it hasn't previously been condensed in such a way at one place that is easy to access and digest. Many books about sex are written strictly from the scientific point of view and not particularly for the layperson in terms that are easily understandable. That is fine for scientists, but there has been a lack of balanced information gathered by someone who is interested in the health/pleasure aspects of sex to improve the understanding and performance of the layperson in terms that they can easily understand. This book should help bridge that gap. I urge you to become exposed to it now, whatever your age is.

The woman's vagina is a wonderful and amazingly complex organ but because they have never seen all of it up close themselves, women don't even know what they are working with. They are as clueless as their mate is. At best, they might have caught a glimpse of the outside of it in a hand held mirror, but all they could hope to see was the outer parts and not in close up detail. The inner parts and the nearly invisibly outer parts such as the Bartholin's glands ports are not visible to them. They don't ever experience a close up view of it during sex and they aren't aware of the symphony of micro movements that their vaginal complex goes through during stimulation and during the orgasmic stage and the letdown phase of sex. Each vagina is unique. They have similarities, but they are also "oh, so different". A woman has to rely on a loving partner to learn her own vagina's precious secrets and then for her mate to verbally convey the secrets on to them.

THE SECRET OF DORMANT RESPONSE CIRCUITS

Women are able to train themselves through a form of biofeedback and micro movement to respond to the individual highly responsive triggers that have always been there, but might never have been activated. This may seem preposterous, but it is actually very true. This fact about dormant and un-awakened response circuits is of paramount importance and it will be discussed in detail later in the book. In most women, at least some of the triggers are never activated so the areas those circuits control forever remain dormant. It takes the recognition that they even exist and then the methodical training of them to become responsive and open the feedback to the sleeping and atrophied parts that they control.

I have spent eight years specifically researching the general subject and a lifetime of experience in learning what questions to ask. Many books have some individual points that are valuable and I have listed some of those books in the bibliography. They are all valuable and you would benefit from all of them. This book is different than any before it because it will give you precise specifics about how you can take the new body of sexual knowledge and learn some new techniques to literally make the sex in the last half of your life even better that it was in your youth. If you are younger, it will give you the head start you need to experience a high level of sexual skill throughout your life if you will open your mind and let the information in. It took my wife and me until age 60 to even realize that dormant circuits could exist.

WHERE DID I GET ALL OF THIS INFORMATION?

The information in this book is condensed from four general sources.

Firstly, by reading books by real experts, studying medical papers and sex research tapes (Sinclair Institute productions and numerous other documentaries), PBS broadcast documentaries, and by reading sex research reports I have learned a significant amount from the numerous and diverse studies by sex researchers, psychologists, and counselors, and have listened to countless lectures on the subject.

Secondly, by observing real couple's relationships over a long periods of time in our business and noticing how life circumstances and menopause changed their attitudes about sex over decades. Unfortunately, some couples found that their post-menopausal sex life was insurmountable and they ended up either feeling unloved, isolated or unappreciated. Some people act on those discontents by divorcing.

Thirdly, by researching a particular form of recorded actual sex sessions using an analytical background. I distinguish that particular form of erotica as being informative and educational as opposed to the huge volume of the staged form of porn that is basal and some of it even degrading. You can find loving sex, casual sex, adventurous sex, edgy sex, kinky sex, and even perverted sex. I looked for the common denominators that made men and women more sexually effective and even more desirable sexually. Surprisingly, thousands upon thousands of couples film their sex lives and put them on the internet for all to see. I was able to observe exactly what specific motions worked best and watched for techniques which were the most consistently effective among a wide range of people. I was surprised at the preponderance of really ordinary and uninspiring sex that most people practice. WHAT REALLY SHOCKED ME WAS THAT ONLY A FEW MEN AND WOMEN HAD REALLY DEVELOPED THE SKILLFUL TECHNIQUES THAT EXCITED REALLY STRONG REACTIONS IN THEIR PARTNERS. The really skilled ones (both men and women) are a rarity. It dawned on me that GOOD SEX REALLY IS A LEARNED SKILL and that it takes some pointed effort to learn how to really be effortlessly effective at sex. Average sex and boring sex come easily and are natural. Is that really the level you are satisfied with or would you rather read this book and study a broader perspective of sexuality and become really skilled? Some very valuable information is out there for anyone with internet access, but it takes a serious amount of time and a methodical approach to ferret it out. There is a definite distinction between luridly watching something and studying it for positive purpose. I have tried to condense key parts of it for you in this book. Like it or not, it is very likely that the internet is where your children and grandchildren are getting probably 90% of THEIR information and much of it is wrong or skewed. Some of it is beneficial, but most of it is either degrading, staged, or downright misleading and they might not have the maturity to discern fact from fiction. Even some of the seriously intentioned material and reports are erroneous. Even the famous team of Masters and Johnson had come to a couple of erroneous conclusions because they were still pioneers in the field. We are all learning as we go forward. Knowledge is in a constant state of change and a constant state of expansion. Long held beliefs can change when new information comes to light. Unfortunately, when surfing the internet, it is too easy for immature minds to gravitate to the sensational rather than the solid and beneficial information.

Fourthly, and just as important as any of the other three sources, the information in this book comes from the first hand personal experience of actively pursuing and attaining a continuingly increasingly satisfying sex life and deeply loving the SAME person for more than 52 years. When I say actively, I mean just that, because it takes a very organized and concerted steady effort to improve your sexuality to the point that you actually control exactly when and how to bring on orgasm. My wife and I both agree that sex is even better now than when we were young when we were chained by ignorance and inhibitions. Both ignorance and inhibitions must be conquered before progress can be made. Sex continues to improve because of the effort it took to gain the information for this book and put it into practice. Who better to learn that part from than someone who has the perspective of actually "doing it" for over fifty years, making all of the mistakes, facing personal demons, concertedly working on new skills, and still having a head of steam to continue on with enthusiasm after age 70.

RIGHT NOW, ARE YOU REALLY SKILLED AT SEX?

Maybe, but probably not! After pondering that question for a minute and being really honest with yourself, you are likely a little doubtful about your skill level.

Don't be insulted by that statement. It is a question you must honestly ask yourself if you really want your sex life to improve with all its rewards. It was a blow to my ego when I had to honestly answer that. I didn't know how little I really knew even though I had made some attempts through the years to learn more. I really hadn't looked thoroughly enough to find out specifically what I really needed to study. I hadn't asked enough of the right questions yet. I was still quite ignorant of a lot that I needed to know and I had to put myself into student mode to learn it.

THERE IS MUCH TO LEARN

I know you will already have a few special tricks that are tried and true, but just for the time it takes you to read this book, open your student mind and allow yourself to expand a bit. We can all learn something more.

If you only walk away with just a couple of important facts to make your relationship better or even save your marriage at any age, the effort will be worthwhile. I MAKE THIS GUARANTEE TO YOU. If you will allow yourself to become a student, put aside your pride momentarily and apply the things you read in this book, your sex life and your relationships in general will definitely improve and your sex life will improve. Is that goal worth the time it takes to read this book and apply it? I also guarantee that you will learn at least ten important facts from this book that you are not currently aware of. Hopefully you will learn many more.

All of us like to think we were born with the innate knowledge to be skilled at sex. How naïve! Did we really think that we could beat the odds and just somehow know everything about sex without an organized effort at learning specific biology and skills? As babies we had to learn to crawl, to walk, to run, then to run faster. Then later decide to go into detailed training for many months if we wanted to become a really good competitive runner. A great pianist didn't get the skill he/she has to be able to play great concerts without years of study and practice. Really good sex is no different.

Practice without some education, or education without some practice isn't nearly as good as education and practice in equal proportions.

JUST A SAMPLE OF WHAT YOU PROBABLY DON'T KNOW

As an example, I will cite that only 14 % of women in one poll had even heard of a G-spot, and almost no one had heard of an A-spot (just recently discovered and documented by an Indonesian doctor), or know how to activate and train either of those areas to produce even stronger orgasms than clitoral head stimulation alone produces. That ignorance also applies to the elusive anterior anal ridge and yet the stimulation of any of these three erogenous areas particularly simultaneously with gentle clitoral stimulation will give catatonic eye rolling orgasms that only a small percentage of women have ever experienced. The anterior anal ridge is the supercharger that starts the fireworks when all else fails. I have never seen anything about this in print or on any scientific documentary or lecture. If you already know about these erogenous zones and think you have nothing more to learn, you are mistaken. There are more than that and there is much about sexual biofeedback and micro movements that will make you and your mate even more responsive and able to sexually communicate. In later chapters you will learn enough about sexual biofeedback and micro movements to make you perform at an expert level.

SEX IS EASY AND FUN FOR THOSE WHO KNOW WHAT THEY ARE DOING

Our Creator gave us a complex instrument that must be studied and practiced to perform expertly and not just use to procreate or to bang out a marginal automatic orgasm. Doing sex without actually studying it is tantamount to a fine pianist standing on the keyboard and simply jumping up and down like a chimpanzee to make music. Actually, watching two unskilled people having sex reminds me of just that---- a chimpanzee jumping up and down on a piano keyboard. Our sexual equipment is much more complex than a piano and in order to learn how to use it really well, it takes study, desire, dedication and patiently applied attentiveness. Most men instinctively have used their member as a jackhammer powered by abundant youthful hormones. At some point in life, those hormones diminish and the jackhammer becomes just one boring tool in the toolbox. A singer who knows only one song becomes just boring and barely palatable even if that one song was fantastic at one time. It just isn't interesting anymore without some variety added to the mix. The same old thing gets boring. A time comes when it is necessary to tune up the old jackhammer and also add some more sophisticated knowledge and some new tools to the toolbox. After all, this is the information age, eh? Guys, the women of today aren't willing to passively accept the lop-sided sex life where the man is the focus and the woman is left hanging and empty as the man selfishly finishes, gets up and leaves her dangling and unfulfilled. Selfishness should be history and should be put permanently into your past. Sexually adept men shouldn't be selfish. Ladies, sex is everywhere and is easily available to your mate, too, if it is you who are the selfish one or if it is you who is the lazy one.

ENTHUSIASTIC IS CRITICAL

You will need to be more interesting and ENTHUSIASTIC than any of the other choices of partners out there that your mate might be drawn to. Complacency and an attitude of taking your mate for granted will destroy your marriage. Shall I dare say it again? BE enthusiastic!!!

If you keep reading, you will find out just how much you and your mate could have been missing and will continue to miss by being complacent or taking each other for granted. Deep down, each of us guys wants to think of ourselves as super studs and women might like to think that they are irresistible because they can just shake their fanny a little and get a man to react. They think they are automatically super divas because we men are such incredibly gullible creatures and will fall all over them. Some women like to think that they just naturally "have it", so they don't think they need to learn any techniques. Some members of both sexes like to think that all they have to do is to just go at it like bunnies with lots of speed and even some enthusiasm, but with little skill. They think of themselves as natural experts. That kind of thinking sets an absolutely minimum standard. That works for procreation, but not for a mutually fulfilling and long term sex life of pleasure and contentment.

LEARN THE MOVES

If the woman just lays there and doesn't really know how to present herself at the correct angles by tilting and moving her hips for maximum stimulation of specific places in her vagina for her own pleasure and for her partner, she is without sexual personality. Only a small percentage of women know this. WOMEN NEED TO KNOW HOW TO MOVE THEIR HIPS LIKE A HULA DANCER, A BELLY DANCER, AND A GO-GO DANCER ALL ROLLED UP INTO ONE PACKAGE. That goes for standing and for lying down. Ladies, that's your first clue. If you are not using your hips in thrusts and gyrations, you have much to learn. That's just to get out of kindergarten in sex school. If the man thinks all he has to do in pump himself up and down with no actual understanding of the several erotic targets he has to actually aim for, nor how to make each one of those magic spots sing for the woman, he is also without sexual personality. Orgasm can occur despite crudeness and clumsiness. Unfortunately that hit and miss mentality is the level that most people have settled into. After you really become skilled, each action is specific and with easier and predictable results for him and for her. Which do you want-- sloppiness and hit and miss results, or would you prefer precision and easily repeated orgasms at a more intense level? Which is it hamburger or filet mignon?

WERE YOU THAT ONE IN A MILLION "NATURAL" ON YOUR WEDDING NIGHT?

How many people really know much on their wedding night? I sure didn't. Did you have the deftness and confidence of a gunslinger at high noon or were you groping and fumbling just to figure things out while trying not to look like a naïve fool? Thinking of yourself as experienced just because you might have had a couple of sexual encounters in the past is just as ridiculous as the pianist expecting to play Beethoven in Carnegie Hall before he/she even learned to play Chop Sticks. You might be playing a Steinway grand piano, so the instrument itself is above reproach, but it sounded like crap simply because you hadn't learned yet how to tickle the wondrous sounds out of that magnificent instrument with the correct knowledge, touch, intensity, and timing. Sex takes all four of those skills to apply to the instrument that the Creator gave to us, but it must be learned. It doesn't come naturally and doesn't come without effort.

WHAT YOUNG PEOPLE HAVE TO LOOK FORWARD TO

Young couples are still dealing with career building, long hours, financial worries, raising a family, and undecided futures and it is really easy to forget that you are on the journey together with your mate and you need to constantly put out the effort to make sure your mate is on the very top of your priority list. I will be so bold as to state that if your mate is not always at the top of your priority list, you will most definitely experience serious sexual problems at some time in your life.

The good news for you is that later in life when you are seniors and when the kids are raised, you have made your mark in the world, and when you are more comfortable with yourself, you can re-bond to a deeper level than ever before with your soulmate. That kind of bond only comes with many years of shared experiences and memories. All of that other stuff is out of the way and it is easier to concentrate on your personal needs. I highly recommend putting out the effort instead of a costly divorce which is all too common for those that don't attend their own sex lives and, even more importantly, the sexual satisfaction of their mate by displaying a loving and giving attitude. It is a certainty that you have grown bored with each other at times or have even briefly thought about strangling each other a time or two. Sexual boredom is common and is normal. It just indicates that there is work to be done. It is up to YOU to make it interesting again. No one else can do it but you.

DON'T FORGET WHO IS THE MOST IMPORTANT PERSON IN YOUR LIFE

Remember your mate, your soulmate, the person that loves you even when they know all of your faults and quirky habits and still loves you in spite of them. Yeah, that same person that has heard every one of your stupid boring stories dozens of times and patiently waits for you to spew them out once more. The person that overlooks the pot belly, your unpredictably flaccid member, your fat rolls, your snorts, your irritating laugh, your drooping man boobs or your saggy woman boobs, your stretch marks, your saggy and wrinkled skin, the tattoo that started out looking like Marilyn Monroe and now looks more like a wrinkled Phyllis Diller, or that long ago cute little butterfly on a tight fanny that now looks more like a shriveled and dying moth undulating on a wrinkled and sagging rear end. That soulmate is the most important person in your life. Do right by them and learn what the hell you are doing so your mate will be deeply satisfied and regularly has the opportunity to experience an even heightened satisfaction of their sexual needs.

Tragically, most people neglect their wonderful soulmate out of familiarity and it breeds boredom and resentment. They let their sex lives load up with psychological baggage that can get so weighty that they look around and find it easy to just substitute other things for amusement and fulfillment. Even worse, they find OTHER PEOPLE for sex and give up on their indifferent and lazy mate who shows little interest in them. YOUR SEXUAL URGES AND DESIRES ONLY DIE IF YOU ALLOW THEM TO DIE, OR IF YOU KILL THEM WITH LAZYNESS AND INDIFFERENCE.

IT'S TIME FOR AN UPDATE

If you are relying on the sexual skills you had decades ago, you are complacent, outdated and need to learn about what has been discovered in the past few years and learn those things which are more available to you now than in years past. The world has changed. This is new information made available and introduced in this book and available for further study through the internet. Anyone that is aware of the specific vocabulary to make the proper searches can access it. I have found that internet searches require a mastery of the vocabulary of the subject you are researching. Most people, young and old alike are also not aware of the same information, despite all of the profuse sexual innuendos throughout our advertising culture and the blatant unfiltered and trivialized sex all over the internet. Many young people know more about some aspects of sex at young ages than their elders did at the same age, but information that is searched under the wrong heading won't answer the right questions. Also, be aware that much internet information comes from the dubious sources of pop culture and is without the balance of many years of experience or the benefit of judicious and critical scientific examination. You will have to be judicious and verify the truth when you run into conflicting information. That was one of my most difficult tasks in researching for this book.

KEEP IT ALIVE

Getting older does not mean that you give up the physical pleasures of sex UNLESS you do nothing proactive to keep it alive. You must be proactive. It is strictly up to you. It is a decision—active or passive. Now is the perfect time to actually catch up on skills and sexual facts that you have not been exposed to. Young people and older people share exactly the same sexual passions and the sooner our culture realizes that, the better it will be for all of our perception of our futures. It is time for you to really get good with your equipment. Older people, get it out, dust it off, and tune it up. Younger people, open yourselves to learning and put in the time to learn the moves.

You younger people, stop thinking you already know everything and get real. You really don't know everything. You will learn much more in life after 50 than you learned before age 50, and if you are just 35, you are probably barely opening your eyes just as I did even if you are astute enough to put out the effort to be aware. This is not a putdown, just fact. I was no different. You won't believe this statement for a while longer, but your traditional "education" can be the biggest factor in limiting your learning any new and different subject. A master's degree in business or another profession doesn't translate to the same expertise in another field, particularly sex, so leave your diploma in your office and leave your intellectual snobbery out of the bedroom long enough to become a student with an open mind. Don't let your ego get in the way of your learning.

SEX FEELS GOOD AND IS GOOD FOR YOU

The fact is, that in the Creator's wisdom, sex is supposed to feel really good and is supposed to make us all want to enthusiastically participate in it all throughout life. The natural response, attraction, and subsequent action is not only normal, but is actually the necessary mechanism of successful reproduction AND mental/physical well-being. Biologically, it would be disastrous if sex wasn't fun or that we grudgingly do it solely for procreation as some belief systems propose. If it didn't feel good and wasn't fun, there would be exponentially fewer offspring. In fact, most of us probably wouldn't exist. That fun doesn't diminish after decades of physical and mental wear and tear, stretch marks, a couple kids, a few extra pounds, some wrinkles, and maybe an infirmity or two. More on that later.

A MORE BALANCED WORLD

If either my wife or I go without sexual satisfaction for more than a couple of days, we become unfit to be around. I hear of people who go for weeks or months or even more without any sexual satisfaction and I can't even imagine how messed up they are. It's no wonder there are so many neurotic and over stressed people and relationships out there. It is no wonder that we still fight so many wars. A buildup of hormones is like being possessed by an evil spirit. It controls you and makes you do things that you would never even consider doing if your sex life was balanced. I believe that a balanced sex life is the most important thing a person can have for good judgement, perspective, and a self-esteem. Sexual release is imperative. SEXUAL TENSION IS ONE OF THE PRIMARY CAUSES OF RESTLESSNESS AND SLEEPLESSNESS AT ANY AGE. Most of the people who suffer from it aren't aware of that causal relationship.

THE LIES WE ARE TOLD

From an early age we are indoctrinated to believe that sex is "not nice", that it is "nasty", or that we should somehow feel guilty for even thinking about it, especially when the beauty of youth is gone. That is even truer of my generation than it is now. Many of us were warped for most of our lives by some pretty twisted views of hypocritical Victorian morality. For example, I was told as a young boy that masturbating would make a person go blind or crazy. From the time we are children, we are taught that we should consciously try to subjugate our natural body chemistry. That way, the numerous forces that hold our society together would maintain their power base over us, and society may continue forward without anarchy. We even conjure a sometimes fictitious and heightened sense of righteous indignation as we become parents and grandparents to demonstrate an air of prudishness to the world. Somehow we have bought into the idea that prudishness rather than understanding is the proper attitude to convey to our children and grandchildren or to the world in general.

KEEP SEX IN ITS PLACE

Who really wouldn't secretly desire a steady diet of moments of ecstasy that we might have first experienced in the seat of a parked car when we were still flexible enough to do a hand spring? Who wouldn't want to continually experience that physical connectedness that comes with the bonding of your true soulmate? Parents, churches, and governments throughout history, mostly for good reasons but some bad, have tried to control our every thought and impression, our standards of sexual normalcy and our sexual behavior. Don't get me wrong, I sincerely believe in boundaries that are conducive to personal responsibility, but I have come to believe through observation that our entire society treats the whole subject of sex entirely backward. It is interesting that many, if not most of those in power only think the rules they try to impose on us don't apply to them and their secret lives. Just watch the news. It is continually full of sexual scandals of the rich and powerful within as well as outside of the clergy and politics.

WE HAVE BEEN TAUGHT ABOUT SEXUALITY IN A COMPLETELY BACKWARD MANNER

It is interesting that almost all advertising uses sex in subtle form and in very blatant form. The message is always that the product being advertised will somehow make each of us more desirable and sexually attractive. Sex in various levels of subtlety is used to hawk everything from food, to cars, to clothing, to houses, and any other number of trifling trinkets. I once heard a Hollywood movie producer state that all leading roles for both men and women are filled by those stars that the opposite sex fantasizes about having sex with (I cleaned up the language a bit). In fact, that sexual attraction even seems more important than the other skills and talents the actors and actresses had otherwise. Sexual attractiveness is what made the producers invest so much money to make them a star to begin with.

Nearly everything in the commercial world revolves around sexual innuendo, but very little SERIOUS communication of actual sexual facts really takes place. It is one of the least discussed topics in open and serious conversation while at the same time being the most insinuated subject on the planet. What a dichotomy, and what a confusing message to send to young adolescents who are still trying to get their bearings in a complicated and duplicitous world! It is the elephant in the room that is continually ignored. I think that is just opposite of the way it should be.

It's no wonder that most people just let their wonderful gift shrivel and even die as a precursor to a shrinking and inhibited personality as they get older. If we were all aware of how sex influences almost ALL of our decisions, we would take it much more seriously. I will repeat a statement made earlier. All human interactions have a sexual component. It sometimes is conscious and at other times we aren't even aware of it. That includes the interchange in the grocery checkout line or the casual "Hello" to a stranger as you pass on the sidewalk. A lot of people wouldn't want to admit this at first, but deep in the recesses of your mind, there is a sexual filter that everyone you meet is subject to in your most private thoughts.

Sex and its intimacy should be one of the most effective weapons we use to ward off the inevitable disappointments we face otherwise in life at any age and particularly in advanced years. We all just need to grow up and begin to give it the serious and open attention it deserves.

Just what makes me qualified to write a book on sex after seventy? As I write these words I have just passed my seventy first birthday with a libido just as strong as, or maybe even stronger than it was when I was a teenager. Secondly, I have been happily married to the same woman for over 52 years and our sex life continues to be more fulfilling with each passing year. Why? We have chosen to put in the time to stretch our skills, face our demons, understand our inner selves, and expand our understanding because we consider it vital to a rich and fulfilling life, particularly heading into our golden years of freedom. ESPECIALLY AFTER 52 YEARS of sex with the same person, that decision is a "must". Are you delusional, you ask? Sex with the same person for 52 years has got to be boring beyond description. "EEEEWWW that is a picture I don't want to imagine!" you say? Maybe not now before you have wrinkles, but someday you will have wrinkles. If you are lucky enough to live that long and lucky enough to still be able to use what you had at age 19, you will need the continuing experimental attitude to make your sex life a vital part of your overall life. Sex is what you choose to make it, and your intimacy is what you choose to make it.

USE IT OR LOSE IT!

Men who are not sexually active have shrinking testicles and shrinking testosterone levels. Women who are not sexually active have dry and thinning vaginal walls as well as several other mental and physical health difficulties or imbalances. The benefits of using it are far better than losing it through distraction, disinterest, incapacity, or laziness. Sexual apathy sneaks up on you slowly like a thief in the night. Sexual apathy will rob you of your intimacy. Sexual apathy will diminish robustness and reduce the length your life. You get out of anything only what you put into it. Good sex takes knowledge, work, mental flexibility, and a determination to want to pursue it. It is a physical and mental imperative to good health, whether you are young, middle aged and especially when you are old. That's why I believe this book is important.

HOW DOES OUR SEX LIFE GO DOWN THE TUBES?

My wife and I started a high end gemstone and designer jewelry business and actively ran it for over 32 years. We had a wholesale business and a separate retail business with clients from very diverse cultures from around the world. During that time, we did business with people from all economic levels. Our retail clients included upper status multi-millionaires, socialites, high level professionals, doctors, attorneys, business moguls, educators and professors, politicians, all the way across the middle class, and all the way down the financial scale to people who work for minimum wages at the other extreme. Our wholesale clients were from diverse cultures all over the world. My point is that we had contact with a wide cross section of people. We were in a high security upper end jewelry and gemstone business, all of which was conducted behind locked doors. We had contact with many of these people for over three decades.

I began to notice that as women AND men reached the menopausal years, their lives took on an entirely different persona due to their perceptions, their religious indoctrination, their culture, their perceived community position, their physical situation, their self-image, and their financial success (or lack of it). Many of them made catastrophic decisions that seriously affected their health, financial position, or personal contentment. Many of those decisions were based on their perceptions and misunderstanding of the paramount roll of one thing. Many of those decisions were based on something related to their sex lives.

This is a book about the subject of sex, so get used to reading that word numerous times. If that embarrasses you or offends you, grow up and start looking into this vital subject in an adult manner. If you just can't get past that, then put this book down, and go read Alice in Wonderland. I will be describing many tried and true, and some new very detailed and very graphic actual sexual practices later in the book that are very prevalent in our society. If you are a true deep down prude or faint of heart, you won't be able to handle it. If you are just a "teeth out" prude, you will be riveted at some of the information that is new to you and even some of the old information that you may just never had encountered in a frank manner. The information has to be very detailed and graphic to really convey the information so it is actually useful and not just another vague and only partially useful innuendo like several books I have studied.

YOU CAN'T HIDE IT

It became evident that it was sex, or even more importantly, THE LACK OF IT, in the lives of many of our clients that began to change them, but not how one would expect. Many times is was about their attitudes toward it. The general subject of human sexuality had always fascinated me and I had always suspected that sex was more important in people's lives than it was commonly perceived. I began to make more serious note of my observations over twenty years ago at about age fifty. At that age I became much more aware of generally how the world REALLY operated---not just how we were told that it did. I became aware of how most of what we were taught throughout life about EVERYTHING is as false or as incomplete as the evening news report. (The really important stuff was never mentioned, and the fluffy stuff and propaganda took the headlines). I began to see how really profoundly our lives are governed by sex. Sex is the atomic bomb of the biological world, and our biochemical hormones, pheromones, and neurotransmitters are the nuclear trigger. People in all power positions know of that powerful connection and use it either consciously or subconsciously to control others. They often use it for their own privilege and as a way to control the rest of us in all of their business and personal dealings.

THE LACK OF SEX REALLY SHOWS

For a few moments, individually picture any number of friends, relatives, and strangers you meet. Notice how their short and long term moods are affected by one thing. That one thing is how long it has been since their last sexually satisfying experience. More crudely put, HOW LONG HAS IT BEEN SINCE THEY GOT LAID, particularly by a partner that was really skilled?

I particularly began to notice the unease and restlessness in post-menopausal women and then noticed the same thing in post-menopausal men. This certainly applies to younger people, too. To put it a bit crassly, how many times have you looked at someone who was acting badly and thought that all they really needed was a good lay? Or better yet, HOW MANY TIMES HAS IT APPLIED TO YOU, but you were too preoccupied, stubborn, or embarrassed about it for your ego to admit it? It is completely natural because it is a widely known fact among sex researchers that hormones build up in the body and that affects moods, judgements, tempers, and attitudes. We have absolutely NO CONTROL over that biological fact. Repressing it through denial only makes the problem more acute. You might partially mask it, but you really can't hide it. The need for sexual satisfaction is evident to anyone astute enough to look for it. In extreme cases where the person is really determined to mask their needs, sexual repression is the result and it can cause serious psychological discomfort and distort ones personality.

A LIFE LONG LESSON

At the tender age of 16, by a sheer fluke of fortune, I worked in a Smithsonian archaeological field expedition on an archaeological dig, and our very colorful 67 year old supervisor named "George" revealed a truth to me one mid-summer day in the hot Colorado prairie sun in a really relevant one liner. As George's small frame slightly bent forward in the hot sun, his deeply wrinkled eyes twinkled and squinted under his flat brimmed hat, and he broke a grin through his very seasoned white, twisted handlebar moustache. He confided to me and a couple of my peers in an authoritatively playful chuckling voice "Sex is the only thing in the world that you can be so impossibly far behind on and catch up in an instant!" The implication of that joke always stayed with me. George had only one good eye (the right one was milky) and his right first two fingers and part of his hand had been shot off. His short frame was slightly stiff and he walked with a bit of a limp. He also had a scar from a bullet wound in his right side. More about George later. I'll tell you how he got the bullet wounds. One is relevant to the subject of this book. You'll love him. George is long gone now, but he was a dear man and full of real life experiential wisdom. George started me thinking that day how really important sex was to our moods and psyche.

SEX IS BIOCHEMICALLY DRIVEN

There is nothing we can do, short of orgasm to even out natural hormonal buildup. How quickly and completely our outlook on the world can change when we have a really satisfying orgasm (or two, or three)! One second you are ready to go to war, and the next second, after a really good orgasm and some close tenderness with your mate, all is right with the world, and nobody wants to go to war. George was right.

Now for the important point---that need for a chemical and hormonal balancing continues all through life well beyond

70—yes, even more importantly, well beyond 70. In later years especially, it can be one of the most connective and comforting things in our lives. Ted Talk lectures are streamed on You Tube on a multitude of fascinating subjects. In one Ted Talk lectures on the internet, it was stated that 54% of those senior between 75 and 85 years old had sex 2 to 3 times a month, and that 23% in the same age group had sex once a week or more. The attribution of those statistics in the talk was the New England Journal of Medicine.

Orgasms and emotional closeness to another human are depression killers. The more we deny the important role of sex in our lives, the more off track we become as we substitute by rationalizing our need for sexual satisfaction into numerous different endeavors. We all have a natural tendency to ignore something that we feel inadequate about and replace it with something that is easier for us. If you feel in any way sexually inadequate, you won't perform at your best. Diverting natural energy away from sex can have seriously detrimental effects on our perception of the world and on our personalities. Diverting sexual desires and energy to other things has serious long term physical and psychological consequences that magnify with each passing year. It can start in teen years as we feel rejected, or can rear its ugly head at any time throughout life. That diversion of sexual energy can progressively distort our personalities into various degrees of a mental pathology.

DON'T WRITE OFF GRANNY YET

One Jewish diamond dealer to whom we bought and sold unmounted diamonds in our business started a side business which was a home health care business for the elderly. He hired out his nurses to families for varying time frames to take care of elderly semi-invalid patients. He used to relate stories to us about the incidents he had experienced in how elderly people REALLY handled their hormonal and psychological needs. The truth described later will surprise you. The famous sex researchers, the Kinsey team, shook the world by reporting what the real sexual practices of people actually ARE, rather than what everyone had assumed that they were. Everyone was shocked at the differences. One of Kinsey's most startling revelations was that our dear, sweet old grandma had a much greater sexual appetite that anyone wanted to admit. She was an active sexual animal, but it was a secret. Families all over America blushed at the thought of grandma "doing it"--- one way or another. "EEEEWWWWWW---YUCKY"!! Who wants to admit that grandma and grandpa have sex drives, too? If grandpa had any interest he was vilified as a "dirty old man". It was unthinkable that sweet grandma would ever think such thoughts because she made you all of those apple pies. Because grandpa bounced you on his knee and played games with you, the thought of him having any sexual desires was just as unthinkable. I guess that in their deluded state, everyone somehow thought that they themselves were a product of Immaculate Conception.

Like I have previously stated, those needs don't go away in old age, and those satisfactions may be one of the few satisfactions that some of those people have left in life. The fact that sexual activity statistically extends life and elevates the quality of life is an added bonus. The really shocking thing is that the family member's reactions are negative so much of the time, rather than clapping and cheering them on with a hearty "go grandma"! The barbarism that the elderly face because of uninformed or prudish attitudes of some families and of some nursing home staffs is disturbing.

As a contrast to this attitude was the true story about a famous boxer's fifty year old wife who decided to pose for the centerfold of Hugh Heffner's magazine Playboy. Her family wholeheartedly supported and encouraged her decision to pose for the nude layout of photos. She actually became an inspiration to 50 somethings throughout America. For those of you who remember, 50 years old then was considered much older than it is today. When I saw the photos, I was about 35 or so and I thought "WOW"! If this is what 50 is, bring it on! I guess that is when I started to change my perception of what old age was. When my grandma was 50, she still wore those awful lace up high top shoes and rolled down long stockings. She thought and acted old. Looking back in it with more perceptive eyes, I know she was still sexually active in secret because of the slightly detectable twinkle in her eye. Even with those hideous high top lace up black shoes she was still a sexual animal. She was quite a character, she was married and divorced 5 times. (I guess some old dudes thought those hideous shoes were sexy). As a young woman she was approached to be a stand-in for a famous Hollywood star of the silent movies. Today's 70 is yesterday's 50.

SECRETS

A psychologist client of ours came through the outer office door of our retail gemstone business one day after being buzzed through our thick 10 foot tall office door. Our massive entrance door had just pronounced a loud, authoritative, and intimidating "kaathunk" when the electromagnetic deadbolt was remotely actuated to allow clients in or out. She entered and visually scanned our two large John Tann high security vaults, noting the authentic Thompson sub-machine gun with a fifty round circular magazine leaning against an open vault door. Slowly nodding her head up and down and with a small sigh of relaxation, she sat down in the leather chair, she stated, "This is the perfect environment for people to really open up. Your office has all of the key elements that we use in our profession. One feels secure and comfortable in here". The feeling of security and privacy from the outside world engulfed people in that office, and they confided things that astonished us. Sometimes they would open up and volunteer the most intimate details of their lives. People continually came to us for a custom designed jewelry gift for someone dear to them. The recipient could be a husband, a wife, or a lover. We were a couple who obviously worked closely in cooperation. The obvious closeness between my wife and me contributed to their ease by adding an air of "insider" stability, safety, and privacy. Due to the nature of our business, many quite intimate thoughts were revealed as they discussed relationships and sometimes dark family secrets. We patiently listened as they talked. Things were openly discussed as though we were part of their family and that we were not just friends or business contacts. Our discretion was absolute. We still keep in touch with several of those lovely people even today after being retired for over 8 years. They knew that their secrets were secure. Once, even a long ago murder was ashamedly and regretfully confessed to us sans the details. All of those secrets remain secrets. The identities will never be revealed.

It became increasingly evident from many conversations that one's sex life had more to do with one's day to day happiness and long term happiness than almost any other factor in life. It seemed as though the sexual component was a major factor in skewing many business, financial, and emotional decisions. It slowly became obvious to me that those decisions were biological hormones talking. Sometimes they outweighed rational thinking to a tragic end. So strange that the subject of sex is so taboo that it is almost never discussed seriously and openly. Yet, every corner of our lives is pervaded with tantalizing insinuations using sex as the messenger with sneers and giggles. How immature and hollow! After years of observations, I decided that it was time that someone spoke frankly and unabashedly about what all of us want to ask or may yearn to tell openly to an understanding ear, but are restrained from doing so by social and religious perceptions, and by our personal hang-ups. Those perceptions keep us bound to a certain form of intellectual and hormonal slavery that deeply affects our health and happiness.

WHICH ONE OF THESE IS PORNOGRAPHY?

As a teenager I was deeply impressed by an article that was published in one of Larry Flint's girlie mags which were hot properties among those of us from the American Graffiti crowd. One article displayed actual photos of atrocities like a beheading, a monk who set himself afire in a protest, a torturous death by a thousand cuts, and a photo of a cancer riddled lung next to a photo of John Wayne smoking a cigarette. In the beheading picture, the dead man's genitals were removed and his bloody head was placed between his legs as a final insult. On the opposite page in contrast, there was a picture of a very natural and lovely naked woman. There was a caption across the top of the pages which read "Which of these is pornography?" I never forgot those images and the indelible impression that humanity is more obsessed with vilifying something beautiful and natural while allowing by default, the truly horrible pornography of man's destructive violent behavior to his own species. Why? How did we get to be such a warped society? From that day forward, I never viewed the tasteful depiction of the human form as nasty, or perverted, or religiously wrong. I will discuss how we got there as a society in the following pages.

THIS IS THE STARTING POINT

I have stated that this book is not intended to be a scientific study, nor a complete work. There are many books already out there by very interesting and qualified authors that cover many related subtopics regarding sex. Those books are statistical studies, psychoanalytical studies, and self-help books. Each one I have read has been beneficial in some way and I recommend that you also pursue them for the things I don't attempt to cover in this book. There is one kind of book that I haven't been able to find. It is the book that gives you the information that this book has. You will see that several of the ideas in this book are my own interpretations and opinions and I believe I have the right to that because of years of pointed study of the work of experts and of over 50 years of personal sexual experience. I make no effort to scientifically document statements because I provide the bibliography for you to read for yourself if you are so inclined. In addition to that, there is the marvel and curse of the internet. I have already done much of the work for you, but I'm not going to do all of the work for you. It is up to you to augment the compiled information in this book with some of your own searches of specifics that occur to you or that may be of special interest to you. My mission is not as much scientific as it is social. My mission is to aid you in your personal awareness and is for application to your personal life. Simply put, do something about it if your sex life is less that wonderful.

This book is partially intended to make the reader aware of how their upbringing has skewed their perception of realities and adjust his or her attitudes to realize how vital sex is to all of us and how completely it effects our decisions and the course of our lives all the way through our advanced years. My intent is then to provide very specific and graphic details of how some old but obscured knowledge and new knowledge of the past few years can be combined to improve our performance and our attitudes to attain a fully satisfying sex life.

Lastly, I wish to say that I am much more of a student than a teacher. That is the tone I hope you will remember when you read this book. This book is about the systematic observations of a 70 plus year old man who continues to learn and who delights in a healthy and abundant sex life. I fondly remember what passionate sex was like in my teens and twenties. As good as it was then, it is far better now. My wife and I are still living the passion of a teenager, but with the surety and comfort of a senior. You sixty somethings, get ready for renewed passion. You thirty somethings, get ready for a pleasant surprise because you will look back after you read this book and wonder how you could have thought that you had the mastery of your sexual expertise without any guidance. I wish the same degree of fulfillment for anyone else at any age who wants the same contentment that my wife and I enjoy.

DO NOT START READING HERE
BEFORE YOU READ THE INTRODUCTION OR YOU'LL
MISS THE POINT OF THIS BOOK!

CHAPTER I

NATURE'S GRAND DESIGN

Sex is one of our most wonderful gifts from our Creator. How we accept that gift determines whether it is a blessing or a curse to each of us. It is a decision made in our own minds.

This book is being written so that we all might be more aware of our Creator's miraculous gift for a contented life which includes a fulfilled sex life. Long ago, man got his own will and our Creator's will confused. Was the original plan of the Creator to be harmony, love, and understanding or was it to be shame, guilt and discord with himself and his surroundings? Somewhere along the way, man started interpreting what he THOUGHT the Creator wanted for us and started to use his own concepts and interpretations to control others. It resulted in some of those men creating a powerful position for themselves over the rest of us.

I could just as easily entitle this chapter "God's Grand Design", but I think it is more exacting to talk about the biology than about the very individually personal understanding of a Creator.

That is entirely another subject. I look around every day and am utterly astounded by the immense complexity and diversity in nature. My wife and I are animal lovers and have had many wonderful and diverse pets in our lives which we consider as equals and close friends and not as possessions. At times in our lives we have also raised livestock for commercial food production. That included mostly cattle, some hogs, some sheep, and rabbits. We have lived in several locations where we were able to observe wildlife families extensively and in detail over long periods. I am in the process of also writing children's books of numerous true stories of the behavioral studies we have made of both domesticated animals and wild animal families. In observing animal families it is evident and obvious other animals have extended families just like humans do. They are not just dumb creatures just because we are taught to think that they are. After years of observations, we have concluded that all living creatures are very similar, even in their magnificent diversity. Life's great diversity belies the fact that all animals (us included) have feelings, allegiances, and a sense of fairness. They experience love, anger, disappointments, and embarrassment. Their experiences include any and all possible emotions that humans experience. In short, we have seen virtually any human emotion replicate in all other animals which we have observed.

OTHER ANIMALS AND MAN ARE MORE SIMILAR THAN WE HAVE BEEN TOLD

It is not that animals are like us, it is more that we are more like them that we would like to believe. Have you ever thought about the statement in the book of Genesis that man has "dominion" over the Earth? I think it means that Man has "responsibility" over the Earth, not "domination" over the Earth as it is commonly interpreted. Despite what many men think, we are not the boss over nature and we'd better get it through our heads that we need to work along with nature rather than to be bent on controlling and dominating everything around us.

Sex, first and foremost is manifested by a chemical cocktail produced biologically as hormones and pheromones and neurotransmitters. We have absolutely no control over that. All of those biochemicals trigger sexual thoughts and desires. I found an interesting example of this by accident. It can also work the other way around. As it turns out, the very opposite may be at least partially true. Behavior might actually trigger or enhance the productions of the hormones and pheromones.

THE SURPRISE EGG FROM CHICKIE

It has been stated by several experts in the field of sexual study that the mind is the most important sex organ.

Our 16 year old African grey parrot whom we had always assumed was a male, laid an egg after a series of short sessions of interactive cooings and neck feather petting from me. I was the one who accidentally triggered it, not the parrot. African grey parrots are extremely intelligent and are considered by most parrot people to be the world's best talkers. " Chickie" as we call her, has an active vocabulary of over 350 words which she constantly evolves to suit her momentary needs. She uses her changing vocabulary in her own sentences which make sense and are not merely chatter. She commonly negotiates with us in words and sentences for whatever she wants at the time. African Greys typically mature sexually at around 7 years or so. Up until age 16, "Chickie" had shown absolutely no sexual behavior at all until I started whispering some different random cooing noises into her ear and rubbing her neck. I inadvertently awoke something after 16 years because she immediately had a very strong reaction. She started making her own unique sounds, panted heavily, and exhibited a caressing behavior on my ear as she sat on my shoulder. She had never displayed that behavior previously. That behavior became obsessive with her over about 10 days. Then on the day before my 70th birthday she laid an egg. I had somehow triggered her to start producing hormones causing the egg to develop, and she laid her egg. HER MENTAL STATE TRIGGERED THE EGG LAYING HORMONES. I really didn't want her to continue laying any more eggs so I ceased that specific interactive behavior and the egg laying stopped. The physical action that somehow simulated mating mentality and caused her to ovulate and lay an egg. Later, I discovered that a bird mating dance was imitated by the man who helped save whooping cranes from extinction. By imitating a mating ritual dance himself, he helped to excite the females and stimulated them to ovulate and to start laying eggs. He ultimately helped save the species from almost certain extinction. Of course, the males were involved, but his displays helped to jump start the process. I mention this because it exemplified how really complex sex hormone production is and hints that we have much more to learn about it in ourselves and other animals. This observation is a true anecdote and a personal experience. It has not been subject to scientific scrutiny with numerous repetitions and many test subjects. I don't have that much time to devote to just that subject, but it would be a really good thesis for a budding zoology doctorate student. Our assumption as humans that we are the masters of the world is a hugely conceited and delusional perception. I hope that I can live to be 100 so that I can look around and see how pitifully little I still know about the universe after 100 years of life. Each year brings at least double the questions than it brings answers. The more we are aware, the less we find out that we really know. I will always remain more of a student rather than a teacher. There is so much to know.

In watching the mating habits of other animals, it became increasingly more apparent to me that we share many if not most behavior traits with them. We have just refined and secreted our behavior so that we each think our habits and desires are unique, but they are not. We are not superior to other animals, we are just sneakier and more delusional to satisfy social indoctrinations. I will give a few examples of related true stories.

UNABASHED DOGS

Dogs have a wonderful sense of smell. Some researchers say that certain breeds of dogs have a sense of smell that is hundreds of times better than we humans.

I doubt that there is a single person that hasn't had their leg dry humped by a dog at some time or another. Our usual reaction is to try to shame or "shoosh" the dog down so he or she will just stop the behavior that is embarrassing to us although the dog seems to think of it as perfectly natural. Sometimes they are pretty insistent. They are just responding to their hormones and to YOUR hormones. The alternative embarrassment is when a dog unabashedly comes right up to a man's or woman's crotch and buries their nose in it for a good sniff of what pheromones you are producing. I'm not suggesting that we humans should go that far in our behavior, but I am suggesting that we need to get some clues from the rest of the animal world about the reality of the world rather our warped and sanitized version of it.

NAPOLEON AND JOSEPHINE

A legendary story is about Napoleon Bonaparte and Josephine. Napoleon was said to have sent a message for Josephine to not wash until they could be together. Did he just like raunchy smelling sweaty women or was he more interested in the subtle musky aromas of her hormones? We have forgotten as a culture, and have largely forgotten as a species, that our natural pheromones are as much a part of us and are as individual and as unique as our faces.

WHY COVER THAT WHICH IS NATURAL?

We go to great lengths to remove all traces of our hormones/ pheromones and substitute some other synthetic "smell good" substance. It is a multi-billion dollar industry. The interesting thing is that the industry spends millions of dollars attempting to reproduce the attraction chemistry that our own bodies produce naturally and for free. As a side note, one recent study has revealed that members of the same family have pheromone smells that are deemed undesirable to members of the same family. The researcher's conclusion was that it was nature's way to insure genetic diversity and discourage inbreeding. Most test subjects found that they were sexually disinterested or even repulsed by the pheromones of close family members, even though they were tolerant of their body smells otherwise.

HOW HUMAN HORMONES AND ANIMAL HORMONES ARE SIMILAR THE HORNY DOG STORY WITH MELISSA AND DAN

I will start some further examples of hormone and pheromone effects with the story of Melissa and Dan. (The story is true but the names are fictitious). They were a couple we had known for many years. I had worked with Dan at different times over several years, and we were good friends that visited back and forth to each other's houses year after year. Melissa displayed the typical restlessness and at times the extreme irritability of a post-menopausal woman. One evening, she and Dan came to our house and came into our kitchen and sat down. Before she could get out a sentence, our little dog suddenly attacked her leg with the fervor of a Jack the Ripper. Legally it would definitely have been considered a molestation or attempted rape if a human had done it. Our little 15 pound spayed female mutt dog latched onto Melissa's leg like a magnet with all the enthusiasm of a crazed buck rabbit and proceeded to make mad love with Melissa's leg. Her tongue (the dogs tongue, of course) hanging out as she rhythmically pumped and panted. Prying her loose from the grip she had on Melissa's leg was tricky at best. The dog was lost in her passion. The dog was a spayed female, and again I will stress that Melissa was post-menopausal. Why such a severe reaction, particularly from a spayed female dog and on a post-menopausal female target?

After that observation and many other observations of both people and other animals over the decades, I have concluded that post-menopausal women are dealing with an atomic cocktail of unpredictable and out of balance hormones that would drive anyone crazy if they didn't know anything about what was happening to them. I began to develop a real compassion

7

and sympathy for those women and their difficult situation. That understanding and sympathy, as much as anything else, prompted me to write this book. The book is sincerely is an attempt help all of those ladies and their husbands to understand their trying situation and learn to use the information in it for enhancing their mutual pleasure and mutual harmony

THE HORNY BULL STORY WITH BONNIE AND CLYDE

Three years ago an elderly couple who were rather recent friends visited us on our small retirement farm. The woman was 68 at the time and her husband was 71. We will use the fictitious name of Bonnie and Clyde. Clyde had long since given up all forms of sex (he probably never knew about more than one form), but it was apparent that his wife Bonnie was not ready to do that. She still had nature blessing her with a steady supply of hormones, out of whack as they might have been. She showed her continued interest with many subtle and covert clues and musings interspersed into general conversation. Her frustration and nervousness were also apparent to everyone around her except her husband. As doctors can testify, many elderly men become fixated on their bowel function and their prostate. Doctors have told me that in some men, it serves as their substitute for their lost sexual proclivities. Clyde was one of those old men who was fixated on his prostate. Many post-menopausal women also use numerous things as substitution for satisfying sex without even realizing it. Bonnie still had strong hormone and pheromone production which I could actually smell.

I had recently had an extensive series of medical treatments called "chelation" to combat a case of combination cadmium and lead poisoning. One of the known side effects of the treatments is a very pronounced olfactory awareness and an acute sensitivity to all smells. It seems to come and go intermittently and is not necessarily a blessing. (There are a lot of really bad smells out there). Anyway, I could smell Bonnie's rather potent natural aromas. We had all gone out to the pasture so they could see the Angus cows and our fine 1700 pound registered Angus bull. Our bull was a sweetheart and he was a very docile creature. He was used to close contact with humans and relished being petted with a fan rake. When bulls and many other male animals smell pheromones and hormones, they raise their heads and wrinkle their noses in a very distinct way to better sniff the air to find the source of the smell. The bull wrinkled his nose, sniffed the air and made a beeline for Bonnie who was sitting on a 4 wheeler near me. Of course she was pretty alarmed at having a 1700 pound bull heading deliberately straight for her and sniffing all around on her. She winced, closed her eyes, froze and didn't know what to do. Since I could also detect the subtle smell, I knew what was happening and I went over to the bull and diverted his attention long enough to get her out of the pasture and far enough away to prevent any problem. I realized that human hormones are similar enough to those of cattle to elicit a sexual response.

Bonnie and Clyde were very religiously oriented even to the point of fanaticism, so I didn't even attempt to say anything to her and her husband as to why the bull was really interested in her. It would have embarrassed her. Her overall behavior was typically of a very frustrated and nervous woman. It would have been obvious to about anyone that what she had needed for a long time was some sort of sexual release and satisfaction, but her religious beliefs couldn't allow her that realization.

She was in denial, and her husband was completely oblivious. What a shame for Bonnie. She will live her remaining years as a frustrated and denied woman. Actually, I have noticed this situation that sexual frustration and tension go hand in hand with many very religious post-menopausal women. Some of them seem to be in a conflicted mental catch 22 situation and really don't know what is happening to them. That brings me to a very personal story from my own family.

A PERSONAL TRAGEDY

My parents were married for over 25 years and they had what I would call a fairly average relationship. Each loved the other in many of the ways that are probably typical in most people's lives. As menopause approaches and gets its meat hooks into a person, much of their rational thinking tends to go out the window if they aren't aware of the symptoms and of the devastation that can result.

My mother began to be fixated on fundamentalist religion to the point that she believed she was getting revelations directly from God. One of my mother's revelations was that she could no longer live with my father as a wife by direct decree from God until my father bowed down and accepted her newfound version of fundamentalist religion and started going to her church regularly, with all the other commitments both financial and otherwise. In other words, she was withholding sex and essentially using it as a weapon, but in her eyes she was only doing what she believed God was commanding her to do. My father had the typical faults of most humans, but was a good man in most ways. Her decree was devastating.

My mother had had some events in her youth which were traumatic and she suffered some guilt that certainly wasn't hers to bear. She had been molested by her father as a young girl and that had resulted in at least one abortion. That was in the 1930's. At that time the entire situation was even more unthinkable than it is now. In addition to that horrible history, she suffered further guilt when my parent's firstborn daughter was stillborn. My mother thought that her stillborn child was God's retribution for the fact that she had been regularly molested as a twelve year old girl and had been forced into an abortion. As if that wasn't enough, when my older brother turned six, he was riding his new bicycle in front of our house, was hit by a speeding truck, and was dragged for over 100 feet. My mother saw it happen and ran to get to him. She held his limp body thinking he was dead while waiting for the ambulance.

My brother's resultant partial paralysis lasted over six months. His very slow recovery lasted over the next five years. She was a very responsible mother, and of course she blamed herself at least partly just like any parent would have. I can see why she felt some guilt, but her own innocence was obvious. This is a nightmare that could happen to anyone. She was haunted her entire life by those events, and it resulted in the destruction of my parent's marriage, even though they never actually got divorced. Mother could deal with all of the tragedy in life up until the time she went through menopause, but then the things that she used to be able to handle as a daily routine became acute and in her mind required severe solutions.

Looking back it seems that a better understanding of menopause itself would have lessened the extremism of the hold her out of whack hormones had on her. She had that same restlessness that I noticed so commonly in other menopausal and post-menopausal women over the years. My grandmother had confided in me that my mother was a very interested sexual being prior to menopause and that she had changed like night and day at the onset of menopause. When she gave up sex according to her new belief system, I believe she simply drove herself deeper into conflict. It was certainly devastating to my dad who committed suicide in desperation at age 49. I look back on it all as a terrible tragedy that could have been prevented or at least made easier with informed and frank discussions about the role of hormones that we don't have any control over. Actually, let me be more precise. With awareness and understanding we do have some control over their management and a more enlightened attitude about their effect on us. I believe that the correct understanding is attained through a balance of education of the role of hormones and a lifelong functioning sex life. I will go so far as to say that when a person's sex life stops, they become more and more unbalanced in other ways. Part of a person dies when their sex life is ignored.

OLD BUT STILL VERY SEXUAL –ERECTILE DYSFUNCTION ISN'T THE END

The next true story is about another client, Vera and Anthony (true story again but false names). One day they were in our office, and among many other short topics discussed, the subject of elderly care came up and I related a story to them that the diamond dealer I had previously mentioned had told us about earlier that day. He had just gotten a call from one of the homecare workers in his employ in his second business which was homecare for the elderly. The worker had called him for advice on how to handle an 80+ year old woman who was using things she could reach to masturbate with. The elderly woman was masturbating to orgasm repeatedly which gave her great relief and satisfaction.

He related that this behavior was not uncommon especially among his women patients. His answer was for the worker to discretely monitor her safety when she self-pleasured, but not to interfere unless it appeared that she was going to hurt herself somehow. What she was doing was completely common behavior and the only thing odd about it is the perception we all seem to have to think that someone who is elderly could still want to "do it". When I told Vera about it, she came back with a series of stories about her knowledge of incidences of the same thing and of active sexual interplay in senior homes that were relayed to her by friends in that business. I became aware that an active sex life doesn't automatically terminate as we age. Unfortunately, open society seems to pigeon hole seniors into the stereotype of sexless creatures. You younger folks should be aware of the sexual needs for your parents and grandparents for their sake and also for the correct perspective for yourselves as you advance through life for your understanding of yourselves.

It appears that many of us actually murder our sex life by inattention or transference to other things either consciously or unconsciously. Vera and Anthony were in their late sixties or early seventies at that time. The even more important thing my wife and I observed in that conversation in that as this subject came up, Vera was smiling, animated and definitely into the conversation. At the same time, Anthony looked down slowly and shyly and unconsciously made his way to the far corner of the office while looking down almost ashamedly. I'm sure he was oblivious to his automatic reaction. It was obvious that Anthony had erectile dysfunction and, to him, his sex life was already over. His expression told it all. NOTHING IS FURTHER

FROM THE TRUTH. His sex life was not over, but because Anthony was unaware of an important fact, it was over in his mind. Erectile dysfunction is an open door to a whole new world of sexual satisfaction to anyone who is informed and interested. The sad thing is that few men are aware of that fact. Erectile dysfunction does not prevent men from having an orgasm as potent as ever and does not prevent them from also satisfying their mates. They just need some new techniques.

A COMMON MISTAKE

MEN WAKE UP!!! I don't know why it is that men seem to feel that their entire manhood and personality is determined by whether they can still "get it up". Newsflash men --- ERECTIONS DON'T MATTER. There is much, much more to a satisfying sex life for you AND for your partner than your sacred erection. MEN REGULARLY HAVE HIGHLY SATISFYING ORGASMS WITHOUT ERECTIONS. Erectile dysfunction is just a good excuse to start learning what you should have been learning when your erection was your signature, your pride, your sense of manhood, and your primary ego identity. Several studies show that from 1/4 to 1/3 of all women don't orgasm during intercourse anyway, but they usually do have orgasms from alternative stimulation instead. That is one of the most commonly quoted sex statistics in print. Men, your "member" isn't nearly as deft as other tools you have anyway. Basically, your precious erection has more in common with the jackhammer that is used to break up concrete that it does to a finely tuned sensitive instrument that it takes to finesse a woman to a controlled A-spot, G-spot, U-spot, or clitoral orgasm with secretions of hormone laden sex fluids. The release of those fluids and orgasm instantly brings a good measure of balance back into her life, a stronger and healthier vagina, and also restores some balance into your own life. Men, get over thinking of your penis as the center of the known universe.

YOU BECOME HAPPY BY MAKING YOUR MATE HAPPY

If Momma isn't happy, you aren't going to be happy either. To the well informed man, an erection shrinks from the dominant focus to a much lesser role in female satisfaction as the proper focus is placed upon the skillful manipulation of the female erogenous areas to produce all of the four distinctly different female secretions that rebalance her psyche so both of your lives can remain in balance. The secretions of those fluids is critical for the full benefits to the female. When, sometimes through excruciating patience, you can skillfully learn to coax her through ascending levels of arousal by caressing the erogenous buttons you already know about AND THEN add those others you will find out about in later chapters in this book. Some of this stuff is still a mystery to gynecologists and is a mystery to much of the medical community according to many articles of ignorance I see published on the internet by a few doctors who, by now, should know better. Even highly educated and well intentioned people are sometimes woefully ignorant of certain things because their particular education and experience didn't include other pertinent facts. They are sometimes laced with ignorance and won't let themselves learn because of their intellectual and educational snobbery. Some doctors are still denying the existence of Skenes fluid, stating that it is urine. That is tantamount to saying the Earth is flat. Many gynecologists have little understanding of effective sexual techniques because their field isn't sex itself and all of its pleasures. Their field of study and knowledge is the human reproductive process and treatment of pathology, not sexual pleasure or sexual techniques. Knowledge of the reproductive process does not translate to knowledge of the sexual pleasure techniques.

Thanks to Kinsey for researching the real sex habits of humans, thanks to the behavioral biologists who over many tedious years have documented the sex habits of the broad kingdom of animals and plants (yeah, plants have sex lives, too), and thanks to the people that most of society loves to vilify. Those are the people who actually film and publish real sexual encounters in such a way that it can become a study and not just a form of entertainment. Among those belittled and vilified for publishing what is commonly referred to as "pornography", there are those who also publish material worthy of study and it is there that some of the most significant information is actually available. The difficulty is that a lot of pure trash and fakery has to be sifted through to find the small percentage of worthy information, but it simply isn't available anywhere else. I have tried to condense some of that important knowledge so that you don't have to do it yourself. I am continually surprised at how much knowledge increases if you keep an open mind, even after you think you are already pretty well versed on a given subject. I have perceived new nuances for the first time even though I had studied the same material several times before. The subtleties are where the gems of discovery are.

CHAPTER II

SEX AND HEALTH

There are many health benefits to those who practice an active sex life. Some specific health benefits of an active sex life continue through life and far into old age are as follows:

Longer life
Better emotional balance
A more even tempered wife
A more even tempered husband
More contentment in all of your relationships
More intimacy with your partner
Physical benefits such as a reduced risk of prostate cancer for men and less chance of heart disease and stroke for men and for women
Reduction of restlessness and irritability
Less aggression and more tendency to compromise during disagreements
Continual re-experiencing the pleasure of orgasm promoting a better sense of wellbeing

with something to look forward to with a corresponding drop in cortisol

A much lessened chance of divorce which can be financially and psychologically devastating, particularly late in life

An overall balancing of hormones in the body which promotes the body's automatic process regulation mechanism

A thickening and strengthening of the vaginal wall

Resumption of vaginal lubrication

The return of more numerous and stronger orgasmic contractions

Less fault finding by both partners which is always a trigger for conflict

This is so important that I will say this one again with specifics:

Men who ejaculate 3 times per week or more have a 40% less statistical rate of developing prostate cancer (reported in AARP magazine). This is due to a buildup of one particular form of testosterone that if left unchecked will cause prostate cancer. In another unrelated study of male cadavers, 100% of men over age 80 that had died from any causes, also had some degree of prostate cancer. I don't know about the sexually active live men compared to the sexually inactive ones. The study didn't cover that.

There is at least a strong suggestion at this time that the flow through of estrogens in sexually active women also lessens the incidence of some types of breast cancer for them.

Men with enlarged prostates notice an opening effect of the

urethra right after ejaculation to allow for effortless urination for many minutes after the ejaculation.

Testosterone laden sperm ejaculate is an anti-wrinkling agent and some women use it on their skin. Testosterone is absorbed quickly through the skin, either internally or externally through the skin. It is also an aphrodisiac for women. Sex experts will tell you that women require a small amount of testosterone in their hormone mix to become aroused. Once the cycle is renewed, it continues to perpetuate.

Close your eyes and remember some of your first sexual encounters in youth. How would you like to feel like that again? You can and you will if you are willing.

I have alluded to the fact in some anecdotal stories in Chapter 1 that sex is one of the most important factors in overall mental health and outlook. I believe that many mental health issues arise from either a denied sex life or an "interrupted" sex life. I mean interrupted as some factor or person being introduced into a person's life to cause them to view sex as bad, warped, as a medium of control by other people as a group or by another person, or a medium for the self to use sex to manipulate others.

THE HEALTHY ALTERNATIVE

The healthy alternative is that an individual is exposed to learning about sex in a loving, sharing, caring, natural, uninhibited, non-sensationalistic, and in an emancipating manner. I believe sex should be treated as a normal and wholesome thing and should be seen as a biological necessity. Unfortunately our society is full of all of those factors that send all of the wrong cues to all ages from little children to older adults. I believe that the way some fanatical religions are taught, that they are one of the major factors in warping the wholesomeness and natural plan in our Creator's design for a fulfilling life. I doubt that guilt and fear are the proper way for us to develop into mentally and physically healthy adults. There are a lot of fine religious people in the world that have pure motives. I consider myself to be akin to them. They really try to live a life of fairness and goodness. There are also many very unbalanced people out there that use religion as their own personal whip to control others and they attempt to influence others to become as unbalanced as they are themselves. They usually are unaware of their manipulation. They are spiritual vampires that suck the joy of life out of anyone they can indoctrinate. Some of them claim to receive divine edicts directly from God which they think gives them the authority of infallibility in their interpretations. Some warped practitioners of various religions are responsible for some horrible travesties, all in the name of their religion and their surety that they are following their God. Read the book entitled "The Dark Side of Christianity" available from booksellers. Follow the atrocities around the world committed by any number of religious radical groups in the name of their religion. Also spend some time studying history of monarchies, power hierarchies, and the origins of religions and how they all interrelate to control the masses of people. Much of what is taught by some Christian churches bears little resemblance to the Christ that I know. There is nothing that is potentially more dangerous than a person who really believes that whatever he does is the will of God. Religious fanaticism is alive and well all over the world under the names of several different religions.

THE LIES WE ARE TOLD

As a teenager, I personally had been convinced that most girls were riddled with syphilis or gonorrhea as I was growing up due to the campaigns by "well meaning" government official programs and publications. These films were originally targeted at GI's, but then were shown in sex education classes in schools. I even thought I would go to hell and burn in eternal damnation if I dared to think any of the thoughts the "church" deemed filthy and vile. We were told that masturbation would make you go blind or crazy and that it would rob you of the energy to do anything productive in life. All that false information did in my life was to create unnecessary conflict in my formative years. Those conflicts weren't resolved until years later when I started to realize the real hypocrisy and mixed motives of those who wanted to retain the reins of power. My father-in-law, a good Christian man of good motive, used to have a saying that I thought was very wise. He used to say "A lot of people get their own will and God's will mixed up!" Not to single out any particular organization, but fundamentalist Christian churches and the Catholic Church are legendary for their leaders who preach one set of values and then violate them in their personal lives. The same goes for other religions as well as for most politicians. Not all, but enough to make note that maybe we should be looking more directly to our Creator for guidance rather than the self-appointed middlemen. All of this underpins mental health.

DON'T LET THE BAGGAGE CONTROL YOU ANYMORE

Let's get back to "Sex after seventy". All of that religious baggage is a large part of why many older people shut down sexually in later years. Add to that, the baggage of a bad or abusive marriage or two, some screwed up kids, some extra pounds, some wrinkles and sags, some financial woes, a physical limitation or two, a few personal failures that diminish self-esteem, some buried but deeply hurtful comments by others, and the uncertainty of old age with limited resources and you get a list of priorities that could easily put sex at the bottom.

George

Remember George from the introduction? He had only one eye and had the first two fingers and half of the palm of his right hand shot off. I promised that I would tell you how he got his bullet wounds. Those hand and eye injuries were accidentally self-inflicted when he foolishly leaned over a shotgun and it discharged when he was a young man as the wild American west was waning. He also had a bullet scar in his right side from being shot as he climbed out a window. He had said to me with a chuckle through his white handlebar moustache and a squinted grin "She told me she wasn't married! Turned out she was lying!" He had already experienced most of those things we associate with advanced age, but he was still vital enough at 67 to be able to joke about sex. George didn't let the baggage hold him down. Did I mention that George held a high position with the most prestigious museum in the United States (Smithsonian). He was a self-educated man who was very much at home in a used book store but also equally at home on field expeditions camped in a tent for months at a time in primitive conditions or in a high level meeting of sophisticated minds. It was a common sight to see George engrossed in a nonfiction book on any number of subjects. He could recite the Gettysburg address from memory and also could recite the Declaration of Independence from memory.

He epitomized that rare combination of a self-driven man who prized education and direct life experience in equal measure. Any time we drove to the nearest town from the field excavation for supplies in the U.S. Army Corps of Engineers carryall van, George made a beeline to anyplace that sold used books. He always spent a significant amount of his pay on stacks of used books to take back to camp to read by Coleman lantern after a day of labor of mapping the grid of the daily archaeological and paleontological finds. George was the epitome of a well-adjusted and healthy sexy senior citizen that any thirty something could aspire to. He was a "can do" sort of guy. George was one of the best balanced people I have ever met, and when I knew him at age 67 and 68, he was as full of life and enthusiasm as a teenager. He always had a sense of humor.

DON'T GIVE UP---ALL AGES HAVE CHALLENGES

Why do some young people just give up on their marriages rather than really work on them when they hit a bump in the road? The physical, psychological, and financial costs of divorce are devastating.

Why do some elderly people just shut down and others get a second wind sexually as they age? I believe it is really quite simple- ATTITUDE!!

You only get out of something what you put into it. In the initial re-awakening, sex takes a lot of effort. It also takes a lot of patience. The rewards sometimes are punctuated by periods when not much seems to progress. This information is from my own personal experience. Sometimes I had questioned whether the effort was worth it.

When my wife had her first really good G-spot orgasm, it was evident that it really WAS worth it. She had always had clitoral orgasms, but neither of us had known about how uninformed we really were. Much advancement has occurred since then and that level just became one of many enhanced skills for us. Also, make no mistake about it, it takes the commitment of both people in a partnership. Giving up is easy, but we are all faced with a choice of making the best of what we have or of succumbing to failure and accepting the false idea that we have already lived our best day.

It is easy to allow life to beat us down. I choose to expend the effort and the considerable patience to obtain the rewards and I convinced my wife to have the patience to put out the effort. I commend my wife for being cooperative and working on new techniques. Remember that the reward is a longer life as well as a much more pleasant life.

A LESSON FROM A SOCIALITE

A wealthy socialite client who came in where I worked a few years before we started our own business. She was high enough up in the socialite ranks that she had everything a person could want in life. She was pretty distraught at turning fifty. At that moment she felt her youth was gone and that it was downhill from there. Then a wonderful thing happened—you know --- one of those epiphanies that we all have once in a while. Her next thought was the alternative---"I could be six feet under instead of merely turning age 50." She never mentioned the fact that she felt old at fifty after that realization. Instead, she saw her glass as half full and that she still had much to look forward to and she actually became a better person. I was about 33 years old at the time and I learned from her lesson. I have since thought many times that I had just become awake at age 50 and have learned more since 50 than all of the years leading up to 50. Experience certainly has its advantages. We live in a culture that idolizes youth, but a guarantee to you that your sex life will be better as a senior than it was when you fumbled around in your youth if you will put the effort into it to make it so. Those of you who are thirty somethings have many wonderful times ahead of you if you keep an open mind and constantly work at improving your skills. When you read the rest of this book, you will have the information to make seemingly unworkable things hum like a well-tuned machine. By the way, for those that don't already know it--- women have stronger, and longer, orgasms than men and women also ejaculate varying amounts of prostatic fluid during the best forms of orgasm (remember, there are several forms). Men, get your mind off yourself and dedicate yourself to learning to coax the best orgasms from your mate. Put aside what you thought you already knew and learn about your wife's vaginal geography. There is a section devoted to vaginal geography later in the book. Trust me, it is more than you think. She will reward you in multiples. Remember the golden rule---"do unto others"---That philosophy does work. Erections are optional for the pleasure of either party. That is a really good thing because in our society over 30 million men have erectile dysfunction and the erectile drugs don't work for many of those 30 million men.

AN IMPORTANT LESSON FOR MEN AND FOR WOMEN

This brings me to another anecdotal story. Michael and Ester were in their late 70's and both of them were vital and fun people (true story, names changed, etc.). They were always both lovable and aware people. One day Michael confided a secret to me that I wasn't aware of at the time. He told me that a "soft on" works just as well for his pleasure as a "hard on" used to work, and that he had adapted. He uses alternative means to satisfy his lovely and willing wife, and she does the same for him. They are in their late eighties now and I still detect that spark in their conversation. They are deeply in love and they still live happy and fulfilled lives. Go Michael and Ester!!!

THE MONEY FOLLOWS THE HEART

There is another health benefit from sex that I will address that isn't immediately apparent, but is one which I have observed over the years to be critical. Our financial health can be seriously compromised if any of several factors are present. Being in the high end jewelry business, my wife and I witnessed the long term changing of spending patterns of many individual clients. The kind of articles we designed and sold weren't sold for chump change and some very significant gifts changed hands costing many thousands of dollars. In observing the spending patterns of specific individuals over a period of two or three decades we could detect where the heart was for the gift giver. We watched as some couples courted, married, and progressed through aging processes and changing priorities. What I am getting at is the tendency for people to either grow together over the years, or to get less enchanted with each other as years passed. The usual pressures of life and raising a family took their toll on some of them. In middle age, several began to be less committed to their spouses and got involved with another person. I know from personal experience that it takes continued active and conscious commitment from both parties in any relationship for it to flourish. One of the first manifestations of a deteriorating relationship is when gift giving starts which is not for the spouse. We had watched as several clients went through this phase of life and sometimes with seriously negative financial results. It usually started when the wife got so distracted by the kids and by social obligations that she didn't properly prioritize her mate at the top of her list. Over time, things became so skewed that her husband felt low on her list of priorities. Likewise, it started by the husband looking elsewhere, focusing on maybe a fresh secretary or business acquaintance, or by the Type "A" husband becoming so embroiled with the office or the business that their attention put their wife at the wrong position in their own priorities. Anything which weakens the attraction bonds between couples WILL have negative financial health consequences. Unrecognized, it will sometimes lead to the financial devastation of a divorce. Divorce is one of the most financially devastating things we can experience.

Financial stability of old age is best preserved by preserving that precious relationship you have spent so long building from a young married couple by feeding it as regularly as you feed your dog "Rex". If you don't feed Rex, he will get weak and die. If you don't feed your relationship, it will also weaken and die. Don't get complacent or lazy just at the time when your mate's self-image and your relationship needs a boost.

YOUNG PEOPLE KEEP YOUR PRIORITIES STRAIGHT WITH YOUR MATE AT THE VERY TOP OF THE LIST

It is important for you thirty somethings to recognize that their mate should always remain at the top of your list of priorities and continually act on it all throughout your life. Nothing is more reassuring than an unexpected and heartfelt declaration of your love and commitment and maybe even a little unexpected quickie on the coffee table when you can sneak away a few odd minutes of privacy. I remember how hard that was when the kids were still around.

The older crowd can delight in the fact that the kids are long gone, it's playtime again, and the health rewards alone are worth it. The mutual sexual pleasure is the added bonus. It is obvious to observe that sexually active seniors are significantly more interesting, younger acting and younger appearing that their sexually dead peers. The spark in their eye is unmistakable

TELL HER BEFORE SOMEONE ELSE DOES

Good quality, interesting, continual, and enthusiastic sex goes a long way toward assuring the love that brought you together in the first place grows into an even more respectful and loving lifelong bond. I can even detect with fair certainty when a couple has stopped having sex by observing the subtle body language and micro body language that we all exhibit unknowingly. The lack of an interesting sex life is a nearly certain way to doom a marriage at almost any age, or at the very least, diminish it to a boring standoff. Any effort you put into displaying genuine love and attention for your mate will yield multifold rewards. I am reminded of a saying that the famous motivational expert, Zig Ziglar, used to state in his seminars. "When is the best time to tell your wife that you love her?" ANSWER--"BEFORE SOMEONE ELSE DOES!" You have made the most serious kind of investment when you committed to your mate and just like any other investment, you have to nurture and protect it. If you even lapse for a while, things can get out of hand enough to pass a point of no return. Sex is just that important. There is nothing more satisfying than to look your mate in the eyes during sex and know that they have been with you every step of the way. You feel that deep respect and commitment to them for all of the sorrows, laughter and millions of life experiences that you and only you share together on this planet.

CHAPTER III

SEX AND NORMALCY

I have pondered the question of what is normal behavior regarding sex for many years and I have come to the conclusion that I don't think there is such a thing as a clear "normal". The two exceptional behaviors that I do not think are normal are the following: I do not think that any form of pedophilia is normal and I also do not think any form of non-consensual sex is normal. I think both are dangerous to society as well as the involved individuals. Precisely, I believe that anything that consenting adults wish to do with their bodies in privacy is their own private business and shouldn't concern either the government or religious institutions. I don't believe it is the business of the government, the church, society, or any other organization to involve themselves in anything that meets the above criteria. I do believe that it is the responsibility of government, and the church to identify, prosecute, and incarcerate anyone within their ranks and in the general public who can be legitimately proven to be a pedophile or a rapist.

WE ARE ALL VERY DIFFERENT

The range of sexual preferences among humans is extremely diverse. Kinsey, Masters and Johnson, Hite and a host of many other researchers since have tackled the subject and shocked the public about the gaping chasm between what people REALLY do and what everyone seemed to want to portray to the world. What actually happens is really different than the false face we put on for the rest of the world. Isn't it time that hypocrisy is unveiled? In Kinsey's studies as a model, the identities of the participants of sex studies was protected in such a way that we began to get the first picture of the candid truth and it shocked society. Or rather, should I say that it made society look at its own hypocrisy? Truth is a powerful weapon and the hiding of the truth leads to false conclusions with little hope of overall improvement of humanity. One of the things that I have found to be fascinating is that mankind as a species is exactly the same today as it was 2000 years ago. Man as a species still has the same avarice, greed, and hunger for all forms of power and exclusivity that he has always had. I'm glad to see the sex studies of the past 60 years dispel many of the general misconceptions about what really goes on in people's sex lives.

WHAT ABOUT HOMOSEXUALITY?

This book deals primarily with heterosexual partnerships and how menopause and aging factors affect individuals in reference to their sex lives and general well-being. Although most facts and techniques contained in this book also apply to other groups outside heterosexual relationships, in order to confine the target of this book more precisely, I have chosen to not specifically address those groups separately. I believe that love is love, no matter what the form, and sex is sex, no matter what the form and I don't condemn any particular group for their proclivities. I just want to keep on my subject and my subject in this book is mature heterosexual adult relationships. It is interesting to note that several studies have revealed a much larger homosexual population than was generally thought a couple of decades ago, and that homosexuality is not simply polarized. The research and resource work that I have done indicates that homosexuality is manifest in varying degrees. Many men and women have some tendencies toward it. Some of those people end up practicing bisexuality in some form which might lean toward one end or the other from full heterosexuality to full homosexuality. It seems to be a matter of degree.

As a personal note, some of my dearest friends are openly gay or lesbian and I love and respect them all dearly. It seems as though all of them have a higher sensitivity to honor and to personal feelings than many heterosexuals. It may be due to a thorough self-examination of their own sexuality and the decision to be openly honest about themselves even when they know much of the rest of the world will likely react negatively and vilify them for it. Maybe we should all be that introspective and honest with ourselves.

REPRESSION

What is normal for a repressed person is very different than what is normal for a more open minded person. Our attitudes and beliefs are subject to the specific culture we grew up in, religion, home environment, and peer pressure from friends and from society in general. Indeed, in some societies, sex is the focus of the goodness of creation and is openly practiced and celebrated as naturally as eating breakfast. Other societies attempt to repress it and make it a shameful act that should only be whispered about if mentioned at all. I see the conflict as a core problem in most people's lives at all ages. I see the truth of admitting that sex feels good, is a natural part of life, and is a vital part of overall mental/physical health is the first prerequisite to facing reality.

LET'S GET REAL

Reality is a human perceptive construct of everything that has formed our personality and beliefs from birth. It is a strange thing, because we create our reality for ourselves. We can create a false reality or we can create a real reality. We then filter our experiences through that filter to conclude certain truths or misconceptions and live our lives based on that. It is a constantly evolving thing that continually reshapes and molds our perceptions of the world. At about age 50, I became aware of the critical need to seek for the truth above all else. All else is false and leads one away from deeper understanding of the inner self and of the world. Is there a benefit in feeding conflict into our lives by constantly absorbing mixed messages of guilt from others who would seek to control us? Isn't it up to each of us to seek the real truth about ourselves?

Man started on this planet with a clean slate and with no rules. As more rules and then laws were enacted by those in power through the millennia, each generation carried more of the baggage of all of the twisted thinking of all misconceptions of every generation before us. On top of that we add our own. It is like all of the thousands of laws enacted by Congress year after year. They keep piling up until the law is just a morass of conflicting ideas that are impossible to be in compliance with. Few laws are ever retired, but hundreds more new ones are added every year.

A LESSON IN HOW THINGS REALLY ARE

The lesson about conflicting laws and the arbitrary interpretation of those laws was made glaringly clear to me when the state tax people audited our business one year. This lesson is also applicable if you examine the laws of various religions for conflict and for arbitrary interpretation. The auditor for the State had determined that we were not in compliance with a particular law on page 17 of the State Tax Code Book, but I pointed out to the auditor supervisor that it was impossible to be in compliance with page 17 if you complied with page 35 and that you couldn't be in compliance with both page 17 and with page 35 because they were in conflict. Everyone was automatically non-compliant with one or the other statute by design. That was the perfect example of the conflict catch 22 that we are constantly being subject to in many phases of our lives. The auditors were well aware of the conflict and said "We choose to interpret the law this way in this particular case and if you have an issue with our interpretation, then take it up with your Congressmen---we don't make the laws, we just enforce them!" If we had been in conflict by practicing the opposite position, they would have chosen to interpret the law against us in the opposite direction. It is a no win situation no matter how lawful you acted. The auditor proceeded to bill us for several thousand dollars which my accountant advised us to pay, thereby justifying the tax authority's existence. I was livid because of the unfairness of the legislature in writing ambiguous, conflicting laws and the arbitrary, and cavalier nature of the auditors' attitude, and of the laws themselves. They were purposely written arbitrarily so they could be enforced arbitrarily. I could sense that he was relishing his two square feet of absolute power that the State had given him to enforce the arbitrary law with finality. My accountant said "You can win this if you fight it, but in the end you will lose because they will then audit you every year as long as you are in business and will harass you until they are able to conjure up something with the conflicting laws to keep hitting you with fines and penalties. Just control your anger, shut up, and write them the check." I was furious because it was just unfair when we were doing everything possible to comply with the law. Our accountant was right because after we paid their arbitrary and unfair levy, we were never audited again. They seemed to be placated by stealing several thousand dollars from us. That was a big lesson in life for me. I further investigated the process and found the arbitrary nature of many laws to be very common regarding lawmaking at all levels. There are many government agencies that use conflict and a heavy hand to bend the intent of the law. Why do I tell this story? Conflict is created by many authority figures in government and other organizations on purpose to justify their existence and to take advantage of others. That conflict can be unjust and it can be arbitrarily enforced by any group of people to further their own end. In the case of religions, social systems, sports, racism, regionalism, nationalism, or militarism, conflict can be created by using guilt or by peer pressure and a sense of belonging to convince people to act in lockstep. Again, read your history. Adolf Hitler was a master of using power to control. An individual person might not be effective in any of those realms to change the status quo of the world's big picture, but you personally can change the status quo where it matters most by doing something as personal and powerful as improving your most personal intimacy skills. It is like education, once you have it, you own it, and it is yours alone to control and use as you decide to better your life.

LEARN NEW STUFF

Since the first studies by Kinsey, it is increasingly known that what is normal in sexual practices is expanding simply due to the common knowledge of what others are actually already doing (i.e. the sexual revolution). An uninhibited sexual relationship is achieved only when BOTH partners are open to some experimentation and introduction of previously untried techniques. It is easy to kill the first awkward attempts to try something new with a half-hearted attitude and with no sense of adventure. Women, your mate needs encouragement and continual communication and direct feedback to know what is working and what isn't. It takes directed attention and some emotional risk to employ any new technique, toy, or idea into a ritual that has evolved into a repetitive and uninteresting or boring copycat sex pattern. It takes encouragement and desire for improvement on the woman's part to fuel the intimidated male partner to try something that might not be received well because of tradition, ritual, or boredom. It's easy to not realize how much courage it takes on the other partner's part to suggest and work on something new that will add spice and variety to a couple's sex life. Many of the new things a couple tries don't work at first, but then after patience and repetitive tries, the new technique will become a new favorite and you will have made a quantum leap to a new level of expertise.

A CONTROVERTIAL SOURCE

As I have previously mentioned, a serious but misunderstood source of some very valuable sex information comes from studying the rather new phenomenon of internet porn and sex related sites and blogs in which a vast array of sexual practices is presented for the viewer and reader. Virtually anything is out there. Some is informational and perhaps entertaining and much of it is just narcissistic garbage in my opinion. Much of it is fake. What is garbage or is beneficial is a very personal judgement. I have found that a detailed study of the sexual sessions self-published by couples themselves is immensely valuable in understanding the differences and the similarities in the vast mélange of humanity. That information added to my own rather sheltered personal experience has given me an understanding of human sexuality that I don't think very many people possess.

I don't know the reasons for so many people of all ages filming and posting their most private activities. I'm pretty sure the reasons vary all over the map. Although some do it for money, the vast majority are amateurs and seem to do it for pleasure and because many of them seem to have a need to record and display their intimate encounters for others to see. The real reasons are probably the same ones that your grandchildren post all of the myriads of details about themselves on social internet media. We live in a very narcissistic culture. I do know that my knowledge has benefitted by studying it, so I am grateful to those people for providing a glimpse into the most intimate parts of their lives.

Many things that sex researchers probably haven't even thought of are videotaped or printed with the most matter-of-fact attitudes.

Some with really astounding implications for a studious observer. It is definitely time for the formally educated sex researchers to open their minds and to meet some of the insiders in the erotic/porn business. The result would be some fresh insight about the working of the human mind/body and for a further understanding of human needs and motives. I have observed several specific educational advancements of the "typical" porn presentation and also have gained some realizations about some legitimate human behaviors. You will need to decide what is normal for your life because it is a very personal decision.

A 50 YEAR TRACK RECORD AIN'T BAD

My own personal experience and observations of having a successful 52 year marriage to the same person which seems to be somewhat of a rarity in today's culture has many benefits. I believe that being able to sexually satisfy the same person for over a half century is more of an achievement than conquering each member of the cheer leader squad, or of a female conquering every member of the football team and having numerous one night stands. I personally believe that it is far more challenging to satisfy the same person for 52 years than to satisfy 52 different women in one night stands. Think about it. The "boring" factor has to be addressed in any long term relationship and factors such as respect and love are not the same for casual encounters. Each scenario has its individual set of lessons and my limitation is only experiencing the long term stance. The other perspective would need to be answered by someone else who has had the opposite experiences. If you know any of those, talk to them about it to gain their perspective.

WHAT ABOUT THE OTHER STUFF

Any honest person would admit that they would be curious about the missing "other side" of their own personal experience. The numerous one night stand scenario is a tempting idea for the person who has always had the same partner, but doesn't have the surety and depth of devotion to a soulmate and true partner. I think the mindset of a long term and caring relationship makes for the least stormy and most contented overall life scenario on a practical and religious basis.

PROSTITUTE FOR A DAY

I recall seeing a presentation several years ago about a prostitute who somehow was chosen to give a talk to a very proper crowd of housewives at a tea party or some such gathering. The housewives were riveted by her insights and enthusiastically bombarded her with questions after her talk. It was apparent that the things she had experienced were fascinating to all the housewives, and for the first time in their lives they had someone who could answer some of the intimate questions they were all dying to know about, but had no one to ask. They were intrigued by her expertise and curious about her. They also temporarily gave her a very limited temporary position of acceptance into their little clique and seemed to transcend any prejudice they previously had after she answered some sensitive questions for the women. Porn is the same way. Everyone wants to openly condemn it because that is what we are supposed to do, isn't it? On the other hand, everyone is secretly or maybe not so secretly fascinated with at least some small part of it. It seems that most women secretly would like to know what it is like to be a prostitute for a day, just for curiosity, but would never,

never admit to the fact, of course, and would never really do it. I think that it is pretty normal to just be curious. It's the ones that protest the most who might be secretly the most curious and have a hang-up. You know what is said about those who protest too much about anything!

FOUR VERY IMPORTANT LESSONS

Make no mistake, there is a lot of real diversity and extremism out there and much of it is truly shocking, but the important bits of intimate vital information I have gained there has been vital to my education of reality. I will relay enough to you that you don't need to sift through all of the extremes to get to a few important facts that can seriously enhance your sex lives. I'll give four specific examples here with much more coming later:

1) It took me nearly five years to verify that the G-spot is not just a simple spot, but an area with four distinct locations that invoke a clearly different response.

2) There are also four distinctly different fluids that are secreted from a woman's vaginal complex during different kinds of stimulation. They all have a different color, consistency, smell, and taste. They don't correspond to the four G-spot arousal locations. I don't doubt that there are even more, I suspect even more discoveries will come and it will be as a result of researchers working in unison with some knowledgeable members of the porn industry.

3) The female pelvic complex muscles and nerves work in a sympathetic echoing "feedback loop". In other words, the entire female pelvic complex is interconnected and can be orchestrated

into more deliberate specific rhythms and crescendos than sex researchers had previously thought. With practice, a woman's mate can learn to stimulate various areas with skillful stimulation and coordinate all of the erogenous areas into a flowing symphony.

4) THIS ONE IS THE BIGGIE! The magic rhythm for orgasmic contractions and building orgasmic stimulus is .8 Hertz (just slower than one movement per second), or sometimes can even be a harmonic of that frequency. The feedback loop may be even more necessarily developed in post-menopausal women than in younger women. I'll discuss more on this in Chapter VIII TECHNIQUES. It is extremely important that you understand how important the .8 Hertz rate of stimulation is to be an effective sexual partner.

The internet has made all information available to virtually everyone who can type into a search engine. Part of the skill of searching is to understand the precise vocabulary of the subject you are searching and let one discovery lead you to others like a detective following clues. The next task is separating the falsehoods from the truth. The internet will be used for good and for bad in the future. Those searches give anyone, including children, and anyone else who have any serious curiosity about anything to find other people of like interest so that they can be candid with them and remain anonymous. Unfortunately, there is always a crass side and children's minds are not mature enough to understand the seriousness of the subject, even though they might think they are mature enough. Many things are beyond what immature minds can digest. The things in this book are definitely not intended for immature minds. Even some adults have immature minds. There is nothing about this book that is wrong, or shameful for mature adults, but immature minds are simply not ready for it.

The internet is Pandora's Box and it is open. There is no going back. We will all have to accept reality and accept less of a fairy tale world. This fact is going to alter reality as we have always perceived it and the established order is in for some surprises. We may even have to stop lying to young children about Santa Claus and the Easter Bunny. The internet has made the world a much more serious and imminently threatening place. I see this transition as paramount to the wellbeing of future generations and I don't have those answers. Thousands of years of religious history teaches us that the "forbidden fruit" scenario didn't work very well, but neither does full permissiveness, so there seems to be a center ground of open and honest discussion of real facts that might be a way to communicate from one generation to another in the information age. One thing is pretty certain. Parents should be an active part of the loop.

I personally did no better with my own children than most other parents did, but the sexual revolution has already hit us and the internet has already hit us, so the problem is right in our faces. I believe only small doses of the truth starting pretty young MIGHT help prepare children for the assault on their senses which is hitting them younger and younger by the likes of the MTV crowd, the rap culture lyrics, and the wide array of internet porn which is too easily available to a much too immature audience.

Maybe we should be conveying the difference between love/sex as opposed to disrespecting/degrading sex as it is conveyed in some pop culture and in trash porn. Isn't that really the point? If we aren't proactive, then we will instead be reactive by default. We will be behind the curve with tragic results. Let's just not throw out the baby with the bathwater in our panic. Rational minds must prevail with valid information and controlled emotion.

CHAPTER IV

THE PATH TO UNDERSTANDING OURSELVES

It has been stated by several experts that the mind is the largest and most important sex organ. If that is true, then it follows that our mind and our attitudes or our "assemblage point" as Carlos Castaneda refers to it, is the center of our sex lives and the power doesn't reside in the sex organs themselves. Every attitude or word we absorb from each and every life experience becomes our assemblage point. Recall especially any cutting words you heard as a child that you were stupid, or fat, or ugly. Remember how you felt! A confident, mentally healthy individual can assimilate things like that into an overall picture of "self" and still carry an overall positive self-image. Unfortunately, most of us carry many of those comments deep in our subconscious, building up over an entire lifetime and take them all the way to the grave. They affect our confidence and erode our potential all through life. Those negative comments can come from a parent, a friend, a boyfriend or girlfriend, a bully, a critic, or from any source that has any influence over us. Many times a derogatory comment is spoken in momentary anger, but once it is out the damage is done forever.

WHAT MAKES YOU FEEL BAD OR GOOD ABOUT YOURSELF?

The first order of business toward a healthy self-image is to recall any and all negative thoughts about ourselves and face them one at a time. It is important to remember how they made us feel and actually momentarily relive the pain for one last time as we face it directly and put it to sleep forever. There has never been a perfect person born, and there has never been a person born that could not be mentally devastated by just the right comment from someone intending to control or hurt them. All of us has an Achilles heel. Some people, many of them in the higher social and economic echelons, are consummate experts at boosting their own ego's by saying things to make others feel bad. We dealt with several levels of socialites and wannabe socialites in our business and we saw this disgusting trait on a daily basis. They learn young in life how to manipulate others. They make themselves look tall by figuratively cutting off the heads of others using snide and degrading comments. The best of them are so skilled that you might not even catch them at their game until after they have left the room. Their timing and verbiage is so perfect that they are gone before you can confront them. They love to use hit and run tactics.

Sex, beauty and fashion is the favorite playground of those vicious sorts. Their power is derived from somehow trying to make you feel inferior to them so they can have the control over you. They are experts at ferreting out and exposing their target's vulnerabilities. The important thing is that they gain that control only if YOU let them. They are like a vampire sucking blood and vitality from your personality by diminishing your self-esteem. Your victory over that trap is to know and understand yourself and to be aware of what they are doing. Learn to recognize when someone says anything to you for the purpose of diminishing your self-respect and avoid them like a plague because they are more harmful to you than the plague. You don't need to go toe to toe with them, just recognize their vitriol for what it is and get away from them. DO NOT INTERCHANGE WITH THEM! You don't want or need those individuals in your life. Resolve to remove them from your life and stay away from them. They are destructive and can be dangerous people but they can be very engaging and charming and that is how they get their hooks into you. Watch several videos on You Tube or read some books on narcissism, sociopathic behavior, and psychopathic behavior for further insight.

REAL CONSTRUCTIVE CRITICISM IS MEANT TO IMPROVE WHILE DESTRUCTIVE CRITICISM IS MEANT TO DIMINISH OR DESTROY

Learn to identify whether any critical comment directed toward you is really meant to help you or whether it is a veiled way of diminishing you.

All physically and verbally abusive relationships are based on one or both people in the relationship being in a continuing battle for domination and control. It will always end in either physical or psychological maiming or psychological death of the controlled party by the controlling party.

Healthy sex is only found in a healthy equitable interchange with neither person manipulating or dominating the other. ANY imprinting from any negative experience in our lives becomes a filter through which we view ALL further experiences. I can't stress this enough.

ONE OF THE MOST IMPORTANT EVENTS IN OUR LIVES IS OUR FIRST SEXUAL ENCOUNTER

One of the most important events of our lives is our first sexual encounter. Any sound, any smell, any sight, any thought, any impression, any feeling (love, joy, shame, guilt, pain), and any physical sensation is burned permanently in our conscious and sub-conscious memory and in some degree will affect how we react to sex in every encounter after that. It becomes a permanent filter. The religious attitude and the self-image we had during our first sex encounter sets the stage for either a positive or negative attitude for sex for our entire lives. Everything sexual that happens to us after that is mentally filtered through that first impression.

WE ALL HAVE A LOT OF BAGGAGE

It is safe to assume that we are all pretty messed up and have a lot of emotional baggage. It is very difficult for many people to admit that to their own ego. How do we fix it? I'm no psychologist, but I am a good observer of myself and of others.

As with all problem solving, consciously recognizing and identifying a problem is step one.

Step two is doing something to fix it. It takes both people in the relationship to heal that relationship. It takes dedicated love and patience, patience, patience to openly discuss painful episodes and memories. It requires finesse and sincerity. It takes incredible courage and vulnerability to be the starter of the healing. To get started, it might only require a good true friend, a mate, a psychologist, or a psychiatrist, or even talking to a bathroom mirror which can sometimes show us more about ourselves than we can find in any other place. No cheating and no holding back. Guys, if some mean girl ever made a crack about your manhood, the memory of her ridicule will always be fresh in your mind. Ladies, I'll bet you remember in detail where you were when your man told you your boobs were saggy, or that your butt has dimples and sags lower than the last time they looked, or that you need to lose a few pounds. All of us are flawed and none of us is perfect. Get over it. Remember, everyone is in the same boat here even though some people are adept at making you think that they are the superior one or the perfect one. Their sincerest hope is that you perceive that it is only YOU with the faults and not them. NOBODY CAN BE IN CHARGE OF YOU PSYCHOLOGICALLY UNLESS YOU LET THEM. Don't let them.

BEAUTY IS IN THE EYE OF THE BEHOLDER

Young women are wonderful to behold with their smooth skin, smoothly curved figures, freshness, and contemporary pop knowledge and appreciation and understanding of the latest "in" thing. They are particularly appealing to younger men who are comfortable in that realm. Other things that young people might not understand and appreciate is stretch marks, saggy boobs, wrinkles, some grey hair, and that extra softness that older women sometimes have which are extremely attractive and very comforting to truly mature men. The older guys might be turned off by the lack of dimensional personality in inexperienced and naively youthful women. Those older women are the ones who know the right songs for a mature man. Those wrinkles are merit badges which are backed up by decades of experiences that make a more robustly dimensional personality. Beauty is in the eye of the beholder and beauty is much more than skin deep. Older women have had the years to develop dimension to their personalities. The more mature perception of beauty would likely be quite different to a youthful observer. It is likely that the younger observer is much more taken with flawless skin, a tight body, and surface beauty. There is nothing wrong with any form of beauty and everyone can admire it. It just becomes a personal preference as to where exactly the beauty resides and just how important each form of beauty is.

SEARCH FOR THE TRUTH AND DON'T LET LIES DEFEAT YOU

Our world runs on piles of lies. I believe in truth and in the axiom that the truth will set you free, but the truth starts by admitting the ugly parts and uncomfortable parts of the truth to ourselves. We are all vulnerable and messed up. It is the human condition. We all have physical flaws and we are all psychologically insecure about something. World religions exist because we are all looking for a way to console our self-perceived inadequacies and find our way back to spiritual communion with the Creator. We all have secrets and secret vulnerabilities. If you can face yourself honestly enough to then face your mate to work together on exchanging all of that baggage, you will build a bond that is stronger than any you have ever experienced. The more open and completely honest you both are, the more intimacy you will attain. If you hold back anything, progress will suffer. My wife hadn't been as willing to do this as much as I was for many years, but since she has, we have made steady progress in this area which directly enhanced our sex lives. I know there can be an asymmetrical aspect of this. THE MORE DIFFICULT A SECRET OR PAIN IS TO DIVULGE, THE MORE IT IS HOLDING YOU BACK AND HINDERING YOUR PROGRESS.   .

WE WANT TO REPEAT THE PLEASANT THINGS

Now, we've looked at the half empty glass, let's look at the half full glass. If your mate has a pleasant or ecstatic memory of the last time you had sex, they are going to want to have sex more frequently. Pleasant experiences are the ones we all want to repeat. The more sophisticated skills you develop to please your mate, the easier it will become to engage in pleasant and effortless sex. Also, the best way you can keep your mate and keep them happy is by being a loving, experimental, passionate, enthusiastic, supporting, honestly complimentary, and patient bed partner. If the last sex encounter was an ordeal for your mate, why would they want to repeat it? It's just that simple. Try to replace the memories of any bad experiences with better ones. It is your responsibility in life to make your mate's life as wonderful as you possibly can. It is both giving and selfish at the same time because any sweetness shown to your mate will come back to you multiplied. In every sexual encounter with my wife, I sincerely try to make the present experience the best she has ever had and sometimes I succeed. I do it with a giving spirit. She is always orgasmic, but her orgasms overall are more intense and more varied with an overall freer and less inhibited bearing since we consciously put the time into improving our skills. We both can see much improvement over time. This improvement can come at any age. It is just as relevant for thirty somethings as it is sixty somethings. Sometimes improvements come in steady succession and sometimes in uneven smatterings, but each year is better. You can do the same. This is imprinting on the positive side. The more fun sex is and the more benefits you see, the more you will both want to participate.

AVOID THE RUTS AND DON'T BE TIMID ABOUT EXPERIMENTATION

It is easy after many years to get into a rut and to not be willing to try different things. We did, so I have first-hand knowledge of it. This is probably one of the most damaging traps to fall into. It results in boredom, less and less interest and you just bore your sex life to death. It can become so acute that sex is an ordeal and is something to be endured. There are only so many positions and you've already "Been there and done that, so what's left"? My friends, the human female body is an absolute marvel. It is anything but boring.

There are so many undiscovered things about the female body that we are just now barely starting to understand a little about the most elusive of orgasms, the whole body orgasm. I have only seen five of them but I believe all women are capable of them and should have them. They are quite dramatic with a completely uncontrollable orgasmic quaking encompassing the entire body. We are becoming more consciously aware of the sympathetic resonance of nerve impulses between the nipples, the clitoral root, the clitoral head, the anal sphincter, the A-spot, the G-spot, and the Skene's glands. Add to that the complex vaginal muscles. The missing information and conflicting information is so rampant that some gynecologists don't even know about the pleasurable part of the sexual function of all the parts that they have studied for their careers in a medical way. Their training simply didn't include information oriented toward sexual pleasure.

A HINT OF A MOST VITAL SECRET

Chemical transmitters and receptors are triggered by the precise frequency of the neuro/muscular feedback loop at .8 Hertz and they are primary for advanced sexual response. The temporary momentary life altering effect on the brain of the sexual fluids release during orgasm is profound. In the "afterglow" phase when the altered and calmed psyche prevails for the next several hours, the full effect on the mind/body/spirit can be felt and observed. To me, that is a miracle. The gynecologists are trained to safely deliver babies as a priority with the detailed understanding of the reproductive system for reproduction and pathological reproductive treatment. The joy of sex is studied by people who want to research and experience the pleasures and benefits of sex. A few of those are in the porn business who are at least partially enlightened for a higher purpose are in that category and are making important contributions, too. It's a shame that there are not more of those types rather than the basal types. Knowledge can be and is contributed to humanity by anyone who is observant and who also has sex.

WHOSE FAULT IS IT ANYWAY?

What if my partner is just boring? Oh, so your partner's personality is at fault and it is the same old, same old routine and positions which you are bored with? That is fixable, but that fix starts in the brain—yours and theirs. We'll address that in Chapter VIII.

It's not that I'm really bored, I'm just tired of looking at her grey hair. Then try a wig or some hair dye. If she is gray haired, try some red hair on either or both ends. How about blonde--- never had that -- Hmmmm! Oh, she just lays there and doesn't wiggle and respond enough to suit you? Then learn whatever skills it takes to make her unable to just lay there motionless. Learn how to stimulate her so she does respond. She will wiggle and respond if you know enough about her equipment to make her wiggle and respond. IF YOU LEARN HOW TO STIMULATE HER CORRECTLY, SHE WON'T BE ABLE TO NOT WIGGLE AND RESPOND. Maybe the old dog just needs to learn a few new tricks. In other words, the old dog needs to get off his lazy butt and learn what he needs to know about what he SHOULD be learning. Forget the "jackhammer her with the schlong dance" and learn some new dances. Learn all of the subtle things that allow you to interpret the micro movements she is displaying. Learn a variety of new techniques. Youthful and ignorant exuberance is wonderful, but gets old and boring and unsophisticated after a while when you have missed her G-spot and her A-spot with all of your chimpanzee moves.

Good sex involves some thinking and some learning of finesse after that initial exuberance of youth is gone. Oh, that's not it you say? He's the problem because his Johnson doesn't stand up and dance anymore and he thinks of himself as just half a man? Is part of the problem his perception of a limp manhood? Maybe he desperately needs some psychological support, some enthusiasm, and maybe some experimentation. Maybe he just needs a renewed interest with an offer from you of somewhere different to put it. Maybe he just needs to catch a distant glimmer of that hot little wiggly chick that passionately used to ride him like a bucking bronco until he yelled "uncle". You, ladies will have to be the instigator here. Be courageous and confident.

THE BEST ON THE BLOCK

If his manhood doesn't stand up like a flagpole anymore, read on and also watch enough oral action to learn how to give him the best blow job on the block. (see chapter VIII) The worst that is going to happen is that you will learn something. His happiness and yours depend on it. Each partner's patience and understanding here is paramount because the longer the sex has been diminished or completely absent, the more mental discomfort and awkwardness will be present to overcome. Breaking the ice here could be even more difficult than your first encounter together, particularly if you are inhibited.

WHICH COMES FIRST---THE CHICKEN OR THE EGG?

It is now known that many women and even some men are not initially aroused as much by thought and are aroused initially by actual physical stimulation first and then by thought stimulation after the physical stimulation has already started. When I first learned that, it was a little hard for me to grasp because I had always been aroused mentally first. The reverse is true for many others. The problem for those people is that no erotic thoughts mean no erotic action without prior physical stimulation in the first example. This can be a deal breaker if both partners don't understand the possible difference between them and how they might respond to action first and thought second or thought first and action second. Women tend to need more physical stimulation first and maybe a little tasteful "dirty talk" to get the engines running, and men might need to see a little skin with a little suggestive teasing to light their fire. Somebody has to press the "go" button first.

SLEEP NAKED AND TALK DIRTY

Seeing my mate naked always turns me on. I will make a suggestion here that really makes practical sense. If you are a post-menopausal woman probably having some hot flashes, sleep naked. It will cool you down and you will tend to snuggle more with your mate. That will warm him up by feeling your bare skin and your intimacy will drastically increase. Try it! Guys, the second she starts sweating, move away and don't touch her until she stops sweating. She'll return to normal in a minute or two.

Hearing the person you love saying suggestive things in their own voice is a turn-on for many people. The first attempts at this might seem awkward, but the humor of it and the ensuing interchange easily leads to more serious and erotic talk which can get really steamy.

MISMATCHED SEXUAL APPETITES

Another thing that can lead to a major chasm of misunderstanding is two partners with mismatched libidos. Sallie Foley, MSW and Dennis P. Surgue, PhD suggest in their excellent book "SEX MATTERS FOR WOMEN" state an obvious, but sometimes unidentified problem. They state that the problem of arousal and of great friction between partners can be a high and low libido difference between the partners. Paraphrasing it, the authors further state that a couple usually reverts as a default to the sexual need frequency level of the low libido partner. That leaves the high libido partner high and dry and continually feeling sexually starved. I personally think this is one of the central factors that magnifies resentment in couples especially after several years into the relationship. The subject is never addressed because both partners feel a certain mismatch and even a form of neglect and betrayal. Resentment toward each other for the difference causes a stalemate that is difficult to address because the open line of verbal communication has already shut down. This is deadly to a healthy sex life.

Each person should ask themselves whether this difference in libidos is a factor in any sexual problems that they are experiencing. It is very probable that it is. Share openly with your partner to get to a deep discovery and understanding of both of your own sexual attitudes, and history, as well as an honest assessment of each of your sexual imprints. Be open with each other about your own personal sexual needs, preferences, and frequencies. If he prefers sex twice a week and you need it every day, get that fact out in the open and work out a frequency of having sex that will satisfy both of you. These subjects are most sensitive and it takes considerable tact and determination to open the first discussion. These frank discussions get easier with time and mutual input.

FORGET WHOSE FAULT IT IS AND MOVE FORWARD

To sum this all up, you may know you are both uptight and you both are probably carrying around a lot of baggage, but now you can admit it, so the conversations start and the understanding begins. You talk it over in several conversations (maybe followed by some fooling around in varying degrees) and have some better understanding, but you still are holding onto some secrets. Go with what you have already have accomplished and relinquish difficult secrets over time. Rome wasn't built in a day! Just wade into the water. You can always go farther later. Discuss some secret desires and even get daring and edgy.

Try some things out and get innovative knowing full well that not everything is going to work for you. Some of the time, most women who are older, and some younger women need some form of vibrator to orgasm in addition to other forms of stimulation. Remember that according to many surveys, a significant percentage of women (over 20%) don't orgasm during intercourse, anyway. The vibrator stimulation might be just the trigger to get the sexual thoughts started in the partner who needs that first. Just about any catalogue of things to buy coming to all American homes has several forms of internal and external vibrators and dildos which come complete with internal vibrators advertised. Anything is available online under "sex toys". Sex shops are in most cities and it is not sleazy perverts that go there. All ages, both sexes and widely diverse types of people go there and sex is treated very matter of fact and the transactions are no different than buying a loaf of bread. Get wild and buy three or four different vibrators or dildos. Some are great and some don't work well for many women. I actually had to build or modify the ones that really worked the best because I am the inventive type. The fun for the man is that you get to try each one out and hold it and watch the very interesting action close up. That's fun. One of our old standbys is a $14 handheld vibrator from Walmart with an electric cord (no batteries to wear out at a critical time). Used in conjunction with an erect penis or a dildo for internal stimulation, a good vibrator is a dependable winner.

ATTITUDE READJUSTMENTS ALTER OUR WORLD

A woman will be as sweet pie for the rest of the day the first time her hormones are rebalanced by your loving attention, understanding, and patience. It may be the first time she has felt really loved in a long time. Do you show your daily appreciation for all of the work she does to make your life better? Do that before you have sex. Your only worry is tomorrow and a repeat performance, but now you already know what to do. Onward and upward!

Ladies, that old grump that you wish would just get out of the house and stay gone for a while will be your errand boy and look at you with stars in his eyes if you treat that limp whanger of his to some tender love and care. And, yes, remember it feels great to him whether it is hard or soft and he can orgasm in either state. Nothing makes a man sweeter that an orgasm. Don't EVER forget that. That note is worth putting on the refrigerator with a magnet. Guys, your reminder note could read "I will not be happy unless she is happy"—"Think orgasm---HERS, NOT MINE." Your mate is the most important thing in your life. Act like it every day. I can tell in just a few seconds which couples are having an active sex life by the way they look at each other and subtle innuendos exchanged between them. Among couples with a good sex life, their other problems smooth out easier because all is well on the home front and they are better tempered and patient. The major bumps in the road smooth out to become minor pebbles. Surprise! Surprise! Who knew, Einstein? Duh!

THE EARTHQUAKE MACHINE AND THE FEEDBACK LOOP

I am going to take a slight but a very important detour here to tell you about something that I consider somewhat my own applications discovery and I consider very important to the subject of this book. I stand corrected if anyone comes forward with proof that I was not original in this thought, but I have never seen the interrelation of this basic physical principle applied to sex.

First of all, every object in the world has a frequency that will make it resonate or vibrate. That is the main point here. Don't lose me here because this is very relevant for you to understand.

I have been involved in developing some inventions in the past years and in the research on background for those inventions, I studied one of the most influential men who ever existed. His name is Nikola Tesla and he was responsible for inventing the dynamo generators that run the electrical grid worldwide in addition to dozens and dozens if not hundreds of other world changing patents. He worked for Thomas Edison at one point in his early career until Edison reneged on an important deal that he had made with Tesla. Feeling cheated, Tesla quit Edison and went to George Westinghouse for financial backing to invent and to build the dynamo which is the basis for the entire A/C electrical grid that we use today. Many people think it was done by Edison, but it was not. One of Tesla's inventions was what he called the "earthquake machine" which could literally make things like buildings or bridges disintegrate with a simple process using constructive interference of a specific frequency. It is accomplished by adding a very tiny bit of energy in the form of resonant waves to continue building the strength of a vibration until the building or bridge literally shook itself to pieces. Simplified, he did it by tuning a frequency generator (radio transmitter) to transmit a specific frequency. Tesla simply slowly tuned the frequency of the electrical vibration on his earthquake machine until it matched the natural resonant or sympathetic frequency of the object he was sending the signal to, and then let physics take its course. As the object began to absorb the energy transmitted at its own resonant frequency, the energy kept adding to the energy that was already being transmitted until the object began to sympathetically vibrate and as the energy continued to build, the object simply shattered as it began to vibrate at the transmitted frequency which matched the frequency of the object itself. The object literally shook itself apart. A clear visual representation of the principle can be witnessed when an opera singer breaks a crystal glass by simply singing a specific sustained note for several seconds which matches the natural resonant frequency of the glass. Another example of this is when thousands of sports fans stomp their feet in unison and accidentally do it at the precise frequency that is resonant to the stadium. They have actually collapsed the stadium and caused multiple deaths several times throughout the world in the past few decades.

THE FEEDBACK LOOP OF ORGASM

The human nervous system works the same way with the muscles when an electrical frequency is set up by a continued rhythm of very gentle and rhythmic touch or rubbing. The manual manipulation of nerve endings in the erogenous zones causes this exact phenomenon in the clitoral head, the clitoral root, the nipples, the penis (particularly the frenulum ridge), the anterior anal ridge, and even sometimes in several unexpected locations such as the ear edges, the nape of the neck, or the feet. As the signals generated by the nerves start to build in synchronized frequency of a rhythmic delicate movement, the signal gets stronger and stronger until orgasm occurs. This is called a "feedback loop" of constructive interference. In the human body, the mechanical stimulation on the erogenous area starts a nerve impulse transmission which echoes into other connected erogenous areas and the amplitude or strength of the sensation builds. If the frequency (rhythm) is just right and for a long enough time, orgasm will occur. In humans the resonant or orgasmic frequency is .8 Hertz or just slower than one motion or one touch per second. The phenomenon is electro/mechanical because it involves the nerve pulses and the associated muscles.

THE SEX VERSION OF THE EARTHQUAKE MACHINE

Several machines have been invented which are for the purpose of sexual stimulation and the most effective of them work on the same feedback loop as Tesla's earthquake machine. The vibrating energy is applied to the erotic tissues of the human body, just as any form of intercourse, oral stimulation, or manual stimulation does by reinforcing and gradually building on the previous sensation in a repeating cycle. Basically, all vibrators operate on that principal using harmonics.

It has been documented that some women can even have as many as 30 plus successive orgasms according to the Sybian Corporation who manufactures a sophisticated mechanical stimulator. It is a device that is straddled with interchangeable shapes and types of dildo penetrating the woman and it has separately controllable vibrating and gyrating actions. I have personally witnessed as many as 17 orgasms in the same woman in a ten minute session. I stress again that his machine is NOT a Tesla earthquake machine, but works on the same principal by reinforcing previous stimulation with added mechanical vibration at the same frequency. The machine has control dials which provide a varying speed and intensity of vibrations and gyrations. The dildo portion is changeable with different sizes and also interchangeable with a fantasy dildo form which is made specifically shaped for G-spot stimulation. I think some of the women who use them feel like they have been through an earthquake as they orgasm with one of them. The sensations are produced with mechanical vibrations and not electrical pulses, but the mechanical vibrations from the machine trigger the electrical pulses from the nerve endings which stimulate the woman's internal vaginal erogenous zones as well as her clitoral head and clitoral complex. It is exceedingly effective.

There is another realm of stimulators which use tiny electrical pulses to accomplish the same thing, but sort of work in reverse to mechanical vibrators and stimulators. They are something like a TENS units which are used by doctors to electrically control pain impulses by destructive interference rather than the building opposite sensation of constructive interference. In the TENS units the object is to lessen the nerve impulses to the muscles to diminish or block pain from injuries. In sexual stimulators the object is to do the opposite by focusing and strengthening the neural sensations to the erogenous zone muscles. I have witnessed as many as ten successive orgasms of women using these devices. One of these devices integrates with the electrical output of speaker wires from a CD player so that the signals correspond with the voice of your favorite sexy crooner or the beat of a rock and roll band. The low voltage speaker wires are connected directly to electrodes contacting whatever it is the person wants stimulated. Special electrodes called transducers are placed into the vagina or on other erogenous areas. These units produce tiny electric signals which can create sound in a speaker and send some of the signal via the transducer to the erogenous zones simultaneously. Unpleasant minor shocks can occur if the connections are not just right and possibly might even cause minor nerve desensitization if used at all improperly. I personally don't like them. I am a bit concerned about these being misused by overzealous people in the passion of the moment and some possible nerve desensitizing might occur. However, many people initially thought that about simple vibrators and that has turned out to not be true. You be the judge. I am simply reporting what exists.

In one form of machine, the mechanical manipulation of the nerves of the erogenous zones produces the resonant electrical impulses, and in the other type of machine, a resonant electrical pulse produces the sympathetic muscular contractions more directly. The two types work directly opposite to each other, but both methods work.

I was introduced to the phenomenon of constructive and destructive interference in my 20's while working in the research and technical departments of a corporation that manufactured high frequency coaxial CATV cable for cable TV. The subject always fascinated me and I was delighted to see that it applied directly to a happy sex life. It is amazing how many devices we use every day operate on this physical principle. The homosexual community was the first to apply the electro stimulator devices for prostate massage and the idea went from there to the heterosexual community. Electro stimulation devices were initially used decades ago in artificial stimulation for bulls to ejaculate into a sperm collector for artificial insemination. The sperm from the bulls was then artificially deposited in small controlled doses into prize cows, thereby allowing many more offspring from very expensive bulls. That earned the bull's owner a great deal more money by using minimally controlled volumes of sperm. With the added feature of not having to transport the live bull in the trailer several miles to the cow, transport risk to the bull is eliminated. For a time in my youth, I manufactured some of the parts for those devices to supply to veterinarians. That was in the early 1960's and the thought of applying it to humans for clinical sexual relief was just on the horizon at that time. I have no doubt that both categories of machines will soon be widely applied in the medical field for certain specific health benefits for humans.

THE BIRTH OF HYSTERIA AND THE BIRTH OF VIBRATORS

Vibrators were invented in England in the late 19th century to medically relieve women of "hysteria" which was the politely acceptable contemporary Victorian term for the need for an orgasm. In that day it was treated as a malady which required medical intervention. When the "patient" needed calming down, she was considered "hysterical" in the sense that she was out of control and somewhat delirious. The doctor simply applied the vibrator to the patient's clitoris who was on a gynecological examination table. The patient was properly draped of course and the whole thing was treated as a medical necessity and not something erotic. Previous to the invention of the vibrator, the stimulation of the clitoris was done manually until the doctors started getting carpel tunnel syndrome from hour upon hour of manual clitoral stimulation. "Hysteria" became quite popular after the Victorian women became aware of the treatment, and for the doctor to apply the treatment was socially and religiously acceptable. What was really happening was that the doctor was performing what a massage parlor does, but it was masked as a medical procedure. The first doctor to use a vibrator ran across a device which was used for another purpose. He then applied it to his need for use in his clinic. It has become one of the most important inventions in the sex world accounting for hundreds of millions of dollars annually in sales worldwide and in the early days it gave many Victorian women much needed relief. I doubt that there are many modern women under age 30 today who don't own at least a couple types of vibrators in some shape or form. There are even small travel models about the size of a lipstick tube to conveniently fit into the purse. Some inventive modern women have used the corner of a washing machine on a spin cycle to produce the necessary stimulation for orgasm. As a side note, the word hysterectomy is used to describe the medical practice of the removal of all or part of the female sex organs to reduce or eliminate drastic hormonal imbalances. This is further indication that the regulation of female sex hormones is vital to female health. I personally believe that if all women have an active sex life, there would be less need for hysterectomies.

FROM CRUDE TO SOPHISTICATED

Vibrators later became married to an ancient self-stimulation device for women which was called a dildo. A dildo is a representation of a phallus and they have been found in many different forms in archaeological dig sites from China, the Middle East, Egypt, greater Africa, and North and South American native cultures. Some were made of stone, some from ivory, wood, bone or from any material that was suitable. Appropriately shaped vegetables such as cucumbers, squash, and carrots were used and still are commonly used as dildos. It appears that female self-stimulation has been around for thousands of years. Today, those materials are being replaced by glass, polished stainless steel, various plastics and "cyberskin" silicone/PVC which is a really accurate representation of the real feel of the living phallus in weight, colors, texture and stiffness with just the right amount of flexibility. They are made in all lengths, girths, and configurations, some have fantasy shapes, and some bordering on the laughable. There are also female counterparts of the female pelvic area available and used widely by men. Many of these are molded from real life models, so the representation is uncanny just as some of the dildos are for women.

The pinnacle of the product is a sex doll which is the full size and weight of a human molded with lifelike cyberskin from real male and female human models and fitted with realistic glass eyes, head hair, pubic hair, makeup, or shades of color. These cost in the low thousands of dollars and are available in any body build imaginable. Looking toward the future, it would not be much of a stretch to see interactive robots joined with this technology to produce interactive sexual computer driven surrogates. We are heading into a vast uncharted future. A later chapter deals more about this subject.

CHAPTER V

⬭

THE SEXUAL REVOLUTION— SOME HISTORICAL PERSPECTIVE

This is a short chapter, but could have been one of the longest. I chose to condense it because the discussion of this particular subject could easily fill an entire book and it is just a point that I need to make to fortify why us elderly (nice term for old farts) should be aware of the changing attitudes of the last 60 years of more sexual awareness.

Opinions vary on this, but in my opinion, four main developments have shaped the American attitude about sex far more than any others. They are all very relevant to a book about SEX AFTER SEVENTY because all four developments have set the attitudes of our generation. They all happened right during our most formative years and we must recognize them for what they are so we understand who we are. It is relevant for the 30 somethings to 50 somethings because they are the first generations that the sexual revolution parents produced and the jury is still out on the result.

THE PILL THAT CHANGED EVERYTHING

Arguably, the most important thing that was responsible for the "sex revolution" was the birth control pill. It completely changed women's attitudes and the way they conducted themselves. It didn't exactly happen overnight, but because it gave women more control over the possibility of getting pregnant it was a real game changer. Those women who came to sexual maturity before the birth control pill didn't have the same perspective that those who came up after the pill. The pre-pill group are decidedly still mentally marked from the social stigma of the possibility of getting pregnant out of wedlock, or within wedlock. They are marked deeply clear up into their 60's, 70's, and 80's even though they can't get pregnant now. Their whole being was justifiably constricted by the fear of getting pregnant. That deeply etched attitude doesn't go away easily. The present generation may have difficulty understanding the degree of their attitude because a pregnancy today of an unwed mother isn't nearly as shameful today as it once was.

The birth control pill actually affected the common person far more than it did the upper classes or the lower classes. The upper classes had always behaved as if the rules didn't apply to them and they were socially exempt from much of the effect of having a child out of wedlock. They could just buy their way out of their predicament whether it was legal or not. The lower classes weren't particularly bothered by what other people thought anyway so they just did what they wanted and perhaps without very much guilt or shame. In the upper classes the most serious sin was getting caught or of being indiscreet. It was the indiscretion that was the major sin, not the affair. That was true for both men and women. All forms of sexual freedom were enthusiastically practiced by the rich and powerful and still are today by many of them. Read some about the private lives of Ben Franklin, the other forefathers of our country, the British royal family, the rulers and elite of all foreign countries of Europe, Asia, the Middle East, Abraham of the Old Testament and you will see that the main group left out of sexual freedom was the middle class which really blossomed in America. Read the newspaper tomorrow and there will surely be examples of the latest rich or powerful person being caught with their dangle in the wrong place. The sexual prison of the middle class was self-imposed in their minds because they were brought up actually believing in the teachings of following the laws and the moral code of the church. Much of the middle class really tried to do what they were taught to be morally right. In short, self-imposed restrictions don't statistically seem to be nearly as strong at either end of the economic or power spectrum. This class distinction is a broad generality and should not be taken to be definitive of all individuals. There are certainly exceptions to this generality in all classes.

MORE AWARENESS OF THE FACTS

The second major thing affecting the sexual revolution was the studies by a new field of researchers studying human sexuality. These occurred before the birth control pill, but I listed them second because I think the pill was even more dramatic toward the change in female attitudes As a total population, people weren't fully aware of the Kinsey studies (Sexual Behavior of the Human Male copyright 1948 and Sexual Behavior of the Human Female copyright 1953), but after some of the juicier aspects of those studies made their way into the conversations of housewives in the 1950's, they became paramount. Then a forum developed over several years which connected the Kinsey studies with the development of the birth control pill a few years later and the sexual revolution began in earnest. Later came another groundbreaking study, the Masters and Johnson study on Sex and Human Loving (copyright 1982). The very readable and important book "The Hite Report, A nationwide Study of Female Sexuality" by Shere Hite (copyright 1976) rounded out what I consider the triad of sexual study. Shere Hite uses questionnaire surveys with vastly different perspectives that give us the basis of true understanding of the sexuality of women. Many books followed after that which give unique and important perspectives on sexuality and all peripheral and related studies. Every other book I have read or referenced on the subject has its own unique facts to offer, but I am confining the subject to a fairly narrow examination to benefit specifically the 30 something crowd and the post-menopausal crowd. After the studies began to permeate the culture, women in particular, began to see themselves as more empowered sexual beings as they realized that what they were shamefully doing in secret was actually pretty normal behavior. After the birth control pill appeared and armed with much new information, women could express their sexuality much more freely without a high degree of pregnancy risk. It is interesting to note here that the study on the sex habits of men didn't seem to threaten society nearly as much as the study on the sexuality of women. Kinsey actually lost his financial backing from the Rockefeller Institute and suffered an unfair and serious setback to his reputation when he published the female study. The double standard was that everything seemed o.k. for men to do. To study that set of facts was tolerable, but society nearly came unglued to find out that women masturbated, grandmothers actually had sex in several forms, and Mom may even be actually having an extramarital affair. I guess society wasn't aware that for every male infidelity, there likely was also a female infidelity. It takes two to tango. All of those men out there who were having affairs weren't doing it alone. Of course, everybody secretly already knew that, but it wasn't openly admitted by society. The studies were so valuable for many reasons, but they were conducted so that absolute anonymity was preserved and people in the study really wanted to contribute by telling their true story for the record.

LEGALIZING ANOTHER OPTION

The third development that revolutionized the American sexual attitudes was the legalization of abortion in America. In the 1950's and before, having a child if you were unmarried was a shameful thing that would follow and mark both the mother and the child for life. The attitude for abortion began to soften in the 1960s and that led later to legalized abortion. After legalized abortion, the stigma became less prevalent and it has evolved now to the point that many women actually tout the fact that they are single Mom's like it is almost a badge of honor. Premarital sex became a much less consequential activity in many young people's minds.

THE INFORMATION HIGHWAY--- A BLESSING AND A CURSE

The fourth factor in the sexual revolution is the internet. The internet is the enormous engine that now governs how all information of all kinds reaches almost everyone in the world. I don't think anyone is wise enough to comprehend the long term effect it will have on humanity. One thing is sure, all of humanity will be exposed to all information at a much younger age than we were before the internet. Much of it will be true, but much of it will be erroneous or downright false. Is society ready for it? How will those younger audiences understand and react to things we considered too graphic for them to digest? How will they handle the inaccuracies and conflicting information? We might all be fooled and it could turn out that because of the absence of the "forbidden fruit", sex, the naked body and the entire realm that the church and society is all so uptight and hypocritical about will become just natural to them. Should society focus be the elimination of hatred, greed, and violence in the world instead? Cultures where sex has been celebrated and nudity is the norm have a far more balanced attitude toward it than us "civilized" folks. Would the world be a better and happier place if we all just accepted sex as a natural part of life with personal responsibility, enjoy it uninhibited, be less uptight, and fight fewer wars.

At age 70, I see more need in the world for love, contentment, and understanding. I see less and less of a place for human greed. I see human greed and the lust for power as causing far more destruction in the world than the fact that two people wish to express love for each other through having sex. Could society be fighting the wrong battle? Where is the ultimate equilibrium that is healthiest for the soul of man?

SEX, RELIGION, AND ART

All throughout history, the prevalent sexual attitudes were reflected in art and religion.

If you study the art world, you will see that sculptures, friezes, and paintings going back several hundreds or even thousands of years from ancient India, Persia, Greece, Rome, the Middle Ages, and the Renaissance have copious representation of sex and the nude human body. Many cultures venerated the human body as beautiful and natural. Christianity taught that the human body was to be covered. Exposure of a naked body was sinful and was the seed for immoral acts according to their teachings. As the western religions took hold in Europe, it became necessary for artists to get past the censors of the day to give a religious connotation to anything with a nude or partially nude representation. For instance, a bare breast on the Virgin Mary holding the baby Jesus was acceptable to the church because she was above reproach, and the naked baby Jesus was acceptable and innocent, but a bare breast of another woman was not. (Interesting rationalization). Wings on a naked baby was o.k. because the baby was then considered a cherub and therefore innocent of its nakedness. Judging by the copious representations throughout history of the human nude form, historically man has had a somewhat healthier balance of the morality of the nude human form that we do in America today. It is a very fortunate thing that the Catholic Popes were wise enough to preserve much of that magnificent art from the conquests of Roman Empire and also the Roman artisans in the sub levels of the Vatican rather that destroying it in a rage of religious fervor.

According to a documentary program on the History channel

entitled "How Sex Changed the World", the Catholic Church actually operated brothels between 300 and 500 A.D and also supported other brothels in business relationships. As long as a percentage of the profit money went to the church, the church turned its head. It seems that sex for money was tolerated by the church as long as some of the money ended up in the church's hands. (Another interesting rationalization). Indeed, some of the most frequent customers were the priests themselves, with the nuns actually participating in the daily administration of the brothels. When the Protestant reformation came along, the Catholic brothels waned. I'm not picking on the Catholic Church here, because all churches each have their own hypocritical corners. Sexuality has always been intertwined in all human interchange, but our private and public attitude toward it is fluid with the times.

CHAPTER VI

∽

THE REGRET OF INACTION

It is human nature to put off doing things that we should do and to do the things we want to do instead. That trait gets more pronounced as we age. Our resolve also seems to wane as we age, too, so the combination makes us think that it's just too much trouble to make any big changes. I believe that many marriages of several decades duration have become a stale coexistence and practical acceptance of all of the lost dreams and passions of our youth. It doesn't have to be that way. The moderate boredom and dissatisfaction at age 30 can become a monumental dissatisfaction at age 60 if not addressed.

I have always believed that effective communication is the basis for all understanding. In any relationship with each other, with the world around us, and with our Creator it is imperative to regularly communicate. Whenever we stop communicating in any of those areas, that part of ourselves first goes into a resignation that we are defeated and then we accept a form of death in a part of our psyche. We must continually believe that we are capable of improvement in all parts of our lives.

COMMUNICATING EFFECTIVELY IS THE ONLY WAY

There are a few individuals I have encountered that simply shut down communication and it is deadly to the relationship. In the business world and in the private world, a person who can't or won't communicate has seriously diminished the effectiveness to function. It becomes impossible to make any further headway in any relationship or business deal with a non-communicator and after many years I have stopped trying. It is psychologically too costly.

If you saw something wonderful in your mate to marry them in the first place, it is likely that trait is still in there somewhere. That goes both ways. My wife and I have gone through many momentary cycles of impatience, misunderstanding and miscommunications of intent. We have used a couple of simple rules to rectify anything of contention. We married when we were 18 years old. Statistically, all odds were stacked against us. We had the presence of mind to agree that if things ever began to develop into a stalemate, we would draw an invisible line on the floor and we would walk up to the line and kiss. I know---it sounds really juvenile and corny, but it worked because it was so elemental and uncomplicated. Almost all dispute resolution began with that action. If an issue ever was so critical that we couldn't quickly resolve it, we always gave each other a little space and then we sat down to discuss the real facts behind our position. A frank and rational, non-emotional discussion would follow and that resolved almost all other differences. Because we are all individuals, there will be a few things where there will always be a disagreement, but then BOTH parties have to allow for that disagreement, knowing that in the bigger picture, the love between you is more important than the issue at hand.

THE HIDDEN EMOTIONS BEHIND OUR POSITION
IS THE TRUELY IMPORTANT THING

Sometimes, much more importantly, the EMOTIONS BEHIND
OUR POSITION were where the sore spot was. Sometimes those
discussions lasted for hours. It is interesting to note that the most
disagreements are nothing more than miscommunication or
poor understanding of the emotions involved. EMOTIONS ARE
THE CULPRIT--- the real emotions---the ones we try to hide---
the ones we are reluctant to discuss---the ones that make us the
most vulnerable---the ones that cause hurt feelings---the ones
that cause resentment---the ones that interfere with uninhibited
sex are the core of bad relationships. We must understand them
and recognize them in ourselves and our mates. We seem to feel
that our precious ego is at stake.

The length of conversations of dispute between my wife and
me has diminished year after year until we rarely have the need
for more than a couple sentences of explanation. The years
have taught us how to fight fairly and to express ourselves more
honestly and openly. That is important to a healthy relationship
and a healthy sex life.

LEARN TO ACCEPT DIFFERENCES WITH RESPECT

There are some things that my wife and I have never agreed on,
but we always came to a truce and we are both aware that we
are both fallible. My wife definitely has her own mind. I love
her and respect her for it. We have always used our differences
and similarities to augment each other. We both have always
pulled our own weight and each of us was willing to do more
than our share at the times when that was necessary. We have

always had genuine love and respect for each other and both of us sought a true perspective of the other person's position. We never "dumped" on each other like I have seen so often in bad marriages. Relationships are like a beam balance like you see on statues of blind justice. They will tilt to one side or the other depending on the weight that is placed on each side. Sometimes one side of a relationship is just heavier with work and worries and that weighs down that side of the scale. In successful healthy relationships, any out of balance of sharing the loads is picked up and leveled out by the other partner having the love and concern to share the problems. It is done out of love and respect and not out of duty. The key is that there is enough love, respect and consideration for each other to want to put the other person before ourselves. Here we are back to the Golden Rule which contains the central wisdom of all major religions.

I believe that if every person put as much effort into preserving their marriage as they do by being negative about their mate, the divorce rate would seriously diminish and there would be many more happy people out there. Put the time and effort into rediscovering all of the positive traits about your mate and build on them. Say and do all manner of nice things that will rekindle the attraction that was there many years ago. Remember that you probably have just as many negative things going on with yourself as your mate has. Don't get me wrong, if you are in an abusive relationship, get out of it. Nobody should have to endure that.

BUILDING BRIDGES

What I am talking about here is that you must be proactive in narrowing the desolate and barren space between you. The space between you and your mate became barren when the two of you made it so with petty bickering and stubbornness. Reconnect first by doing the little things like providing an unexpected cold drink on a hot day, by a tender hand on the shoulder and a sweet inquiry about how he or she feels, by a squeeze of the hand and an understanding glance. Do you remember the very first time you held hands and how your heart fluttered or pounded with anticipation at the uncertainty of whether your gesture would be accepted? That is the kind of feeling that will return to you in a short time. That feeling will grow if you are proactive and make it grow. Be lovable and you will be loved. Be despicable and you will be despised.

Indifference is easy but it is the food of fools. If you do nothing, then nothing will happen. You must be the instigator and take the lead. Prepare for many minor disappointments along the way. Remember that you didn't get where you are quickly. It took years. The return road is easier if both you and your mate recognize what has happened and BOTH of you want to fix it. Your mate's surprise and delight that you still care may astound you. Be bold and take the first step and then the second--- just like a baby learning to walk. If you had a car accident at age 60 and had to re-learn how to walk again it is the same thing as relearning how to emotionally reconnect. If you are in my generation, you have a few or even several years of life left and you really don't have any time to waste. If you are in the 30 something group, don't waste the best years of the middle of your life with unnecessary strife.

STOP PUNCHING THE WRONG BUTTONS

My guess is that you know exactly what turns your mate "on", you also know exactly what turns them "off" and you are pretty good at using both buttons. Forget the "turn off" buttons and just resolve NOT to use them—EVER---. Dust off the "turn on" buttons and exercise them regularly. The result will change your entire relationship for the better. You know exactly what irritates your mate and surely you remember what they like. The Mexican standoff that you have defaulted to over the years has likely been a subtle battle of your skill in using the "turn off" buttons to retaliate for your mate's use of your "turn off" buttons against you. Do you remember playground politics in grade school? Don't you think you are really past that stage of life?

A MIDDLEMAN CAN BE USEFUL

As you read this, seriously consider having your mate read this book with you and discuss openly between you what has been discussed on these pages. Discussing the words of a third party allows a bit of distance and a bit of protection when a disagreement needs to be settled. Somebody else to gang up on and blame is sometimes helpful. I gladly offer myself as the third party scape goat. Disagreements can become a habit and actually be the focus of contentious individual's existence. The strife almost becomes their goal. They may even get so they live for the conflict as if it was a game and they are keeping score. The third party (in this case, me as the author) can absorb some of the recirculating animosities and be a common ground for the start of agreement. Even if your mate reads this book and declares "He is full of crap!" Don't give up. Keep being kind and loving and just keep trying. Your efforts and patience will very likely win out in the end if your partner is worth keeping around anyway. If they don't, the exercise will help smoke out a doomed situation and you will be on the high ground.

NO SEX WITH THE EMOTIONAL ENEMY

Why am I bringing all of this stuff up? Really good sex is something that comes AFTER the emotional pathways are in order. IT WILL NEVER, EVER COME BEFORE the emotional pathways are in order.

Compare the picture of two people who regularly show open love, respect and attraction for each other to the picture of two people who are scowling in irritation and boredom and can hardly stand to be in the same room together without verbal digs at each other. I like to look around in restaurants at couples of all ages and notice how engaged or disengaged they are with each other. I know you have seen couples that eat their meals as if the other person wasn't even there. I think that is so sad, because it looks as if they are so bored and disinterested with each other that they are already dead. My wife reminds me that sometimes people might just want to be left in quiet enjoyment and might not want to always be communicating. My answer is that they are communicating their deepest inner feelings without saying a word. Their scowling or blank expressions say it all. Just examine yourself and see if any of this applies to you and your mate. If it doesn't, then you can go on to the next chapter. If you can see yourself in these examples, this is where you need to start before anything else will help you become vibrant and sexually relevant once again.

THE TERRIFIED SOLDIER, HIS LOVE, AND A PROMISE

One day a wonderful old man wheeled his wife into our office and they quickly became our friends and occasional clients. He was a trim, tall, soft spoken, gracious, and loving husband who lived to make his sweet wife's plight in her wheel chair as bearable as possible. He was a bomb bay operator in a B-17 bomber crew in WWII and was a retired military man. His wife had suffered a stroke that had left her nearly fully paralyzed and so slurred in her speech that he was the only one who could understand her. He was patient and loving beyond belief. He relayed a story to us a few months after our initial meeting and as we became more familiar friends. He told of a bombing raid they made over Germany in which flack shells were bursting all around. Suddenly two shells smashed clear through the fuselage of the plane whizzing just past him and also just missing the bombs they were carrying. The flack shells left gaping holes below him and above him and passed well above the plane before they exploded. He wasn't one of those men who bragged about his role in the war. He was just relaying the terror of war through the eyes of a man that was little more than a boy at the time he lived the story, and expressed his gratitude to still be alive. We could detect the fear in his voice as he told his story. His wife had been the sweetheart at home that he wrote to and thought about in order to mentally get through those horrible times. She was the reason he had to live through the terror and she was the person at home to come back to. His love for her was so tender as he reached down to her drawn up hand to lift it and straighten it out enough to put on a beautiful diamond dinner ring that he had purchased for her. "Here Babe, I told you that I would get one of these for you someday", fulfilling a promise of long ago. That is the couple that reminds me of the dedication that we should all have to our mate. A tear wells in my eye as I remember this. It was a very touching moment.

IS YOUR MATE WORTH IT?

Think back at all the wonderful things your mate has done for you through the years on special occasions, in difficult times, and the shared good times. Isn't that the person that you really loved and would like to renew some sparks of passion with? Now think of the times that you were maybe not as understanding as you could have been, were indifferent, unthoughtful, or even downright hateful. While you are both still alive, fix it!! There are no guarantees in life. FIX IT NOW before it's too late and you are haunted by what could have been if your stubbornness and pride didn't get in the way. For a moment, forget yourself and your precious pride and just make this about your mate. Start by making a list of a few things you could make amends for, write down a few things you appreciate and go to your mate and just say it all out loud to them from your heart. Unless your relationship is already truly dead, your mate will respond enough for a new beginning. What have you got to lose? At the very least it puts you on the moral high ground. This is a no brainer. You may soon both start considering your mate before yourself. That's what you both should have been doing all along. That attitude was likely present in the first months or years of marriage, and then something happened. That something began to fester little by little until you realized one day that you were unhappy and, of course, the person that you directed the blame to was your mate. It is easy to blame the other person rather than looking into the mirror, but the mirror is the place where we usually find the culprit that has sabotaged our life. Have the courage to face the mirror.

AND THEN THE E-MAILS STOPPED

I have already said that life has no guarantees. About 4 years ago, I noticed that I hadn't received any E-mails for a while from a particular friend. My friend, Lenny, was a big and burly ex-marine with hands the size of ham hocks. He was a no nonsense and gruff looking sort of guy that said exactly what he thought. To me, that was refreshing in a world where mealy mouths are all too common. After his service days, Lenny had become a merchant marine engineer and had been promoted to Chief Engineer in charge of the maintenance of three of the huge ARCO oil tankers that moved crude oil from Valdez, Alaska down to the lower 48 states. He spent his duty time aboard the ships on their runs. His job was important and he had to keep up with the specifications of literally thousands of systems and sub-systems. It is no job for a fool. The thing about Lenny is that he had a secret. Under that gruff and coarse exterior, a real teddy bear filled his large hulk. Lenny contracted cancer after he retired, but he didn't want his wife to tell anybody about it. One day his wife called us anyway and told us. My wife and I traveled to the hospital in another city the next day to visit him and he was, of course, surprised to see us since we weren't supposed to know. No one had been to visit him. He was really pleased that we were there and openly showed it. It was as if new life was breathed back into him. Lenny liked us both and respected us, and really felt honored that we would come visit him. He had been is pretty bad shape, and I really don't think he would have survived more than a few days. The fact that he did survive seemed to be from the psychological boost for him to believe that two people would drive a distance just to come see him, talk with him, pour him a glass of water, and really be genuinely concerned for him. He hid the fact that, like all of us, he really wanted to be loved and cared for, but just didn't want to show it. His gruff persona belied the tender teddy bear that most of us have hiding somewhere inside. That part of him was touched by our simple display of affection and concern to someone that the whole world thought was as tough as nails. Lenny lived for about 2 years longer and then the E-mails stopped for good, and oh, how I miss them. Thank God we went to see him. God bless you Lenny. I wonder how many of us display that same turtle shell tough exterior while inside we are mostly just teddy bear mush. When our feelings get hurt, rather than say so and resolve the issue, we try to buck up and act tough so we hide our vulnerability. Anyway, back to Lenny. I coined a phrase that unfortunately I have had to use too many times since. THE DAY THE E-MAILS STOP IT'S TOO LATE. Don't wait for the E-mails to stop to fix the problems. Get over yourself and hold out the hand of conciliation and make up for lost time by resolving to replace each unpleasant memory with a better one. That applies both in and outside the bedroom. Your mate IS the most important person in your life. You owe it to them to let them know in very specific terms that you love them in any way you can----over, and over, and over again until the E-mails do stop and then it would be too late.

BE EXPLICIT---NOBODY IS A MIND READER

Tell your mate in great detail EXACTLY what it is about them that you appreciate. They can't read your mind and you can't read theirs. Tell them often what physical traits they have that turn you on. Tell them specifically some of the instances that have occurred throughout your marriage that made you respect them. Tell them how they complete you and bolster your own shortcomings. Imagine the hole in your life that would be there without them and express that realization to them in words. Tell them in precise detail how you feel. Resolve to make the last years of your life your best years full of spiritual and physical love. If you do this sincerely, with heartfelt sincerity while looking directly into their eyes and holding their hand, your relationship will make a quantum leap in the right direction and you will be well on your way to being able to advance your physical love to deeper levels. This step is absolutely vital before anything else can be expected to happen. Men are 80% teddy bears and 20% raw insecurity that needs constant reassuring. The ones that project the toughest personalities are usually the biggest babies with the most insecurities. Women aren't very much different despite all the jokes and discussion otherwise. We all take a risk to bare our true emotions and expose our fragile egos. All of us have had our feelings stomped on many times. Make yourself vulnerable in order to become stronger.

HURT FEELINGS FESTER BUT FORGIVENESS AND LOVE IS FREE

The negative imprints that are caused by hurt feelings can make us into bitter old scowling creatures. We have to dig deep, deep, deep and get into the things that really hurt us the most and are our deepest secrets. It takes further risk and boldness to continue to reach into the depths of ourselves for the fullest understanding of ourselves and others, but the rewards far outweigh the risk to our ego. Love is the one thing that costs nothing to give away. You can give it for free no matter what your physical or financial condition is. The supply of love is inexhaustible because the more you give away, the more you have left. For every single time your feelings are hurt, determine that you will respond with love in return. I don't think this a Pollyanna attitude.

There are a few people I have run into that are unreachable. No matter how nice you are to them, they just don't respond. It is probably because of their own psyche of hurt feelings and negative imprints. I have made it a practice to allow 5 years to deal with each of these rather rare people and if I don't make any headway after that, I walk away and let some other force deal with them because they are out of my ability to understand.

CHAPTER VII

———— ∞ ————

SOME NEW FACTS, QUESTIONS AND ANSWERS

We have addressed the relationship part of a fulfilling sex life, so now it is time to get to what might have drawn you to this book in the first place. The physical side of sex. This chapter lists a few of the rather new information that wasn't common knowledge when our generation was coming into adulthood. Most people of our generation haven't made themselves aware of this information unless they have been active seekers of information through the years to enhance their sex lives.

FACTS

FACT #1

The sexual revolution has spawned a new kind of woman who is no longer willing to silently endure selfishness in men's treatment of them. They are much more knowledgeable about their own bodies and have been exposed to more sexual information than we were and at a younger age. Post-menopausal women are more educated today about sex. They are typically are more prone to sexual experimentation than ever before. Women are no longer willing to be left without sexual satisfaction.

FACT #2

Men are much more likely than they once were to be sexually interested and active into their 70's and 80's today due to the availability of drugs to help overcome erectile dysfunction. Unfortunately most men have a fixation and a dependence on their penis alone to satisfy their partner. The new erectile dysfunction drugs give them a boost in confidence. The macho self-image they feel with their new "stiffy" boosts their personal measure of their manhood. Most women answering surveys say that they prefer a good lover who knows several methods of stimulation much more than those who just thrust their penis in and out in the same old boring fashion again and again. The modern Renaissance man has a box full of tools and knows the precise techniques to use them effectively for their mate's maximum pleasure. Besides just being able to target just the right spot to pleasure his wife during intercourse, he is skilled at oral sex, manual sex, and the use of sexual aids to delight his partner.

FACT #3

Postmenopausal women now have the means easily available to them to obtain and use self-stimulating devices for their sexual experimentation and satisfaction either with or without a partner.

Insecure men are often threatened by this. They shouldn't be, it saves a lot of work for us and actually makes our roll a lot easier. (Remember the doctor who invented the vibrator--- you really don't want a bad case of carpal tunnel syndrome, do you)? Women should be experimenting sometimes on their own, particularly if they are among those who didn't masturbate regularly as young women.

FACT #4

Post-menopausal women have a more open attitude to use self-stimulating devices because of the women's liberation movement and because there have been so many sex study books that have shown what their peers are already doing. They realize that they are normal to want and expect sexual satisfaction. Their attitudes are more relaxed than in previous generations and the self-stimulating devices are readily available to them to purchase from the privacy of their home.

FACT #5

The internet has made so much information privately available with a simple search, that both men and women are able to privately answer questions about any intimate subject. (One caution is that much of the information on the internet is inaccurate or purposely staged or deceiving). Some internet articles and blogs are useful and some are not. It is easy to go down false paths if you rely solely on the internet and don't read some books by sex researchers.

FACT #6----- (VERY IMPORTANT)

Finally, the question about whether there is such a thing as a vaginal orgasm as opposed to a clitoral orgasm has been satisfactorily answered. YES, THERE IS SUCH A THING AS A VAGINAL ORGASM. The famous psychologist, Sigmund Freud, was the first to attempt to explain the vaginal orgasm as a "mature" orgasm. To some extent I agree with his conclusion because some degree of mental maturation and seasoning has to be accomplished in many women to discover and then to train the neural pathways to open up and respond to G-spot and A- spot, and U-spot stimulation. More about this in Chapter VIII which deals with specific techniques. Clitoral orgasms don't require as much "training". Clitoral orgasms are the quick and easy way, but only account for a partial experience. Like a woman once stated to me, "There is no such thing as a bad orgasm!" But then she also stated that didn't know anything about a G-spot orgasm at the time, either. There is such a thing as good, better, and best. Why settle for just good level when you can experience a higher level? There are actually several different kinds of vaginal orgasms. The difficulty is that it is extremely difficult to isolate and stimulate a single erogenous zone without inadvertently calling the whole orchestra into action because all parts are interrelated and don't act alone. The very easy act of stimulating the clitoral head stimulates the pubococcygeus muscle which in turn stimulates the anal sphincter muscle, and stimulates the clitoral root, engorges the clitoral bulbs and Skenes glands. That all unleashes a flood of hormone laden liquids which trigger further contractions, causes mental changes, and completely involuntary changes in all of the smaller muscles around the vaginal vestibule. Just clitoral stimulation tends to train the female to become accustomed to the quick and easy fix. Further training teaches women how to isolate the different erogenous zones and make them work separately or together as desired. Without some further training, she may never learn to go on to experience the deeper and more satisfying form of orgasms involving the specific stimulation of the specific erogenous parts of the vaginal canal even though she may have had many years of experience with intercourse stimulation. She may think that's all there is. My wife and I didn't know about anything further until after we turned 60. What a shame!! You 30 somethings take note. Intercourse alone doesn't train the required erogenous areas of the vagina to respond to a vaginal orgasm. This is where foreplay must be mastered by the male partner. Again, more on this in "Detailed Specific Techniques- Chapter VIII". If internal vaginal stimulation is introduced in several specific areas, some degree of vaginal orgasm will result only AFTER a woman has opened her neural pathways to allow it to happen. Most post-menopausal women will be carrying a serious load of baggage from their upbringing, their societal stigma, and possibly some disappointing or even bad sexual experiences. Those psychological issues MUST be addressed first. They are very likely imprinted with some experiences that have at least partially closed down their neural pathways of response. That is where I think Freud had it right. His "mature" orgasm, that is, a vaginal orgasm, requires the removal of the neural pathway blocks. I can't stress these steps enough. My conclusion after much study and practice, is that in women, there are only various degrees that each part contributes to the overall orgasm depending on exactly where the major stimulus is directed AND where it has been opened to respond with directed practice. In the beginning stage of waking up the neural pathways it is like a paralysis and no matter how hard your first tries are, nothing will work. That kind of control is much easier to learn with manual or hand stimulation by her partner than with intercourse. For example, it is almost impossible for adults to control a sideways movement of their small toe simply due to atrophy of the nerves and muscles that control it. We never use it so it is atrophied. If you don't believe me just try moving your little toe out sideways and see how difficult it is to even establish the neural connection to make it move a small distance sideways. The exact same thing is true of the atrophy of the vaginal erogenous circuits. They must be a discovered, awakened, and then tuned with patient practice.

An orgasm can be let's say, 70% G-spot #2 zone, 20% clitoral head, and 10% U-spot, or it can encompass several other erogenous areas in varying combinations. (SEE BELOW in FACT#7) In short, it can be virtually any combination of the types listed below. It becomes up to the man to provide the encouragement for the woman to overcome inhibitions and to cooperate consistently and long enough to get results, but I can't stress enough how great the rewards are for those that are willing to do it. The critical role of the woman is to be patient, cooperative, exploratory, open minded, and willing to drop inhibitions. That's no small task. It is no less for the man. At the post-menopausal stage, the gender load balance of inhibitions sometimes tends to reverse. Then, men then can be plagued with some degree of erectile dysfunction which is a real blow to his sense of masculinity if he is not enlightened to the many other tools he has to still be a virile pleasurer of his partner. He can't allow his erectile dysfunction to become an inhibition. He may not naturally have the courage to overcome his penis dominated ego and look around for alternative techniques. If he lives long enough, every man will definitely experience some form of erectile dysfunction. At that point it is up to the woman to encourage her mate to get past those feelings of inadequacy and cooperate to gain a broader understanding of the previously ignored techniques and possibilities. A skillful male lover must understand women's physiology and vaginal geography in detail before he has any hope of really satisfying her consistently. Very few men really seem to have that knowledge, but hopefully this book will help and they will be heading in the right direction. A woman must understand the very delicate male ego and penis fixation so that he can develop other techniques which are even superior to the old jackhammer syndrome. Men please note: Most women are far less fixated on your penis than they are with the other techniques you use to satisfy them. We will work on that in a few more pages. Your own reward will follow from a truly satisfied and grateful partner.

FACT #7

Many different types of orgasms have been identified by various names that are not always consistent from study to study. I won't cover some of them because several of them such as mental/ fantasy, exercise, and kissing orgasms are more rare and if they affect you, you already know how to do them. Sixteen various types and kinds of orgasms that I name here are named and categorized slightly differently by other studies, but this list works well for my purposes. They are listed here using my own terminology:

THE KEY POINTS FOR PRODUCING ALL
ORGASMS--- (IMPORTANT)

Orgasm occurs when the stimulus of an erogenous area is at the precise frequency. That frequency for humans is .8 Hertz. Put another way, it is one movement of the finger, the tongue, or thrust of the penis or dildo at the speed of slightly less than one per second. IT SEEMS TO BE AN UNNATURALLY SLOW SPEED AS SEXUAL STIMULUS PROGRESSES TO A MORE HEIGHTENED STATE, AND FOR THAT REASON MOST PEOPLE SETTLE INTO TIMING THAT IS MUCH TOO FAST. Be patient and count out the seconds until you are automatically aware of this all important rhythmic speed or frequency. Remember that magic number of .8 Hertz and when you increase the speed, you should double it to .4 Hertz or slightly slower than a half second per movement. That is the first harmonic of .8 hertz and it is the frequency that shifts the neuro/muscular gears into "high" to get the orgasm rolling down the highway faster until the orgasm occurs. Shifting the stimulation to an in between or non-resonant frequency for very long results in a destructive interference, or a dampening down of the stimulation, although a very brief stopping or breaking of the rhythm for only a second or two, actually sometimes seems to light the afterburners on her jet engine. It sounds complicated at first, but just shoot for slightly slower than one movement per second until you are accustomed to it. All of this is a subtlety that takes some practice.

I list 16 specific types of orgasms, but some studies use different terminology and parameters according to their explanations.

Orgasm type #1--- Clitoral head and clitoral root

The delicate rubbing of clitoral head for women causes a clitoral orgasm. The frenulum area and penis head for men (always with lubrication) causes a similar type of orgasm.

The deeply embedded clitoral, root and vestibular bulbs work with the clitoral head. The rhythmic indirect movement of the wishbone shaped clitoral root and bulbs that partially encircles the vagina at the vestibule are stimulated by penetration of a finger, a dildo, or a penis into the vagina. They attach to the clitoral head to the deeper and more extensive parts of the vaginal complex much like the roots hold a tree in the ground. Movement anywhere around it indirectly stimulates the clitoral head and the neurological ties to other erotic areas. The clitoral root is directly tied to the clitoral head, so a clitoral orgasm involves these parts, too. Most women don't know this fact about themselves, and most of their partners are completely clueless.

The glans, or penis head, of the man is analogous to the clitoral head of the woman. The clitoral head has even more nerve endings than the penis head. Some studies state that the clitoral head has as many as 5000 nerve endings and some studies quote as many as 7000. I have personally never tried to count them and I wouldn't know where to start, but I will take the researchers word for it when they say that the number of nerve endings on the little clitoral head has even more than in the whole male penis head in which the nerve endings are spread out over a much larger area in the head of the penis. I make this point for the benefit of those men who don't understand how really sensitive the clitoral head is. That wonderful button has a concentration of more than ten times the actual density of nerve endings than a penis does in a similar sized area.

Orgasm type #2---G-Spot for women (Named after Dr. Graffenberg who discovered it.)

The Skene's glands corresponds to the prostate for men. There are 4 distinctly different zones on the G-spot in women. Let's call them #1, #2, #3, and #4. Each one produces a distinctly different kind of sensation once they are all awakened. The #1 zone starts at the bottom edge of the pubic bone just inside the mouth of the vagina, the #2 zone is a puffy spot barely inside the vagina behind the pubic bone, the #3 zone is the area slightly deeper into the vagina which is cross rippled in most women, but squarely behind the inside flat part of the pubic bone and is what some studies refer to as the full G-spot, and the #4 zone is about as far as you can reach inside the vagina with a hooked finger, past the cross ridges, but well in front of the cervix. They all respond to very different touches. The correct type of stimulation of the G-spot varies depending on the specific area (#1, #2, #3, or #4). The specifics are given in the next chapter.

It took me nearly 6 years to learn how to give pretty consistent G-spot orgasms of all four types. I'll tell you why when I discuss techniques. In doing so I discovered the 4 separate areas of the G-Spot that give the 4 distinctly different reactions. I have never seen that information anywhere else. Usually, a woman's G-Spot is just considered one area. Each zone of a G-spot orgasm is a separate experimentation. More on that a little further on.

Orgasm type #3---A-Spot

Recently discovered by an Indonesian doctor as a separate erogenous location in women, it is the area on the upper side (or front inside of the vagina as standing) which is between the cervix and the upper terminus of the vagina. WE HAVE FOUND

THIS ONE TO BE HUGELY IMPORTANT. It particularly responds to gentle (not forceful) pressure against the terminus of the vagina in a gentle thrusting motion of a penis or dildo. It is a very deeply satisfying form of orgasm. It has no visibly discernible structure associated with it, so it actually completely skipped detection until recently. Once awakened, is a very welcome addition in itself, or to coordinate with other areas of stimulation. One particularly effective technique is to vary the depth of penetration back and forth between the G-spot zones and deep thrusts which put gentle but firm pressure against the vaginal terminus after the woman has become comfortable with the deeper penetration. Up until its discovery, several medical papers stated that there were no stimulating structures in that area of the vagina and that the deeper half of the vagina had no erogenous capability for the woman. Nothing could be further from the truth. (I wonder how many more things we don't know that will be discovered with further investigation). The A-spot response is VERY powerful when done correctly and at the correct time during penetration and with the proper frequency of rhythmic movements. The degree of pressure and timing are critical. At the beginning of stimulation the pressure against the deepest end of the vagina should be gentle with the penis or dildo and with the pressure increasing very slowly with successive strokes to a firmer pressure using the orgasmic frequency of .8 hertz (slightly slower that one stroke per second). At orgasm, firm to very hard pressure is necessary and usually urgently demanded by the woman, but NOT TOO SOON.

Orgasm type #4--- Anal anterior fornix

An anterior fornix is in the anus on the vaginal side just about the depth of the cervix of the vagina. I like to refer to this as the "pot of gold" because when you find this one and know how to make it really sing with the precise timing and pressure, it is a near instant orgasm and it synchronizes everything else that is happening throughout the pelvic bowl. It is EXTREMELY powerful. That is really shocking to me because I have never seen anything about it in any of the literature on erogenous zones. Stimulated together with the clitoris, the anterior anal fornix delivers a consistent deep catatonic orgasm to the woman and continues past orgasm as long as the gentle stimulation remains. Stimulated correctly in this manner, a woman can be brought to near orgasm and kept there skipping along for long periods just barely under orgasm, usually with her eyes rolling in a catatonic like state. Upon orgasm, additional VERY slow and VERY gentle (and I mean VERY GENTLE) stimulation will continue to maintain a very high level of arousal extending long after orgasm. Sometimes one simple touch in this area will start orgasm. As this area is stimulated it changes drastically in texture in waves, throbs and spasms. It is really something that deserves a great deal more research.

Orgasm type #5---Cervical –particularly, the hard ring of the cervix.

The cervix is round and doughnut shaped in women who have never been pregnant. It is more slotted to differing degrees in women who have at some time been pregnant, or even more slotted in women who have given birth. Pressure or gentle friction directly on or around the cervix is erogenous to most women. Again, correct speed and timing of stimulation here is important. The area all around the cervix is highly erogenous and the face of the cervical opening is also separately erogenous in a slightly different way. The position of the cervix in the vagina varies among women. It is sometimes at or very near the upper end of the vagina and sometimes it is located an inch or two from the upper end of the vagina.

Orgasm type #6---U-Spot

The U-spot is stimulated around the urethra and just barely inside the urethral opening on women. It is best stimulated during cunnilingus with the rough texture of the top of your tongue or very gently with the slight roughness of your fingerprint on a single finger. The U-spot is also directly stimulated during intercourse with penetration at a particular angle and very slow steady strokes. Too much motion seems to drown out the stimulation of the U-spot. It is best to stimulate the U-spot during the buildup phase in foreplay for some diversity. Use the magic orgasmic rate of stimulation of .8 Hertz.

Orgasm type #7---Multiple orgasms in a continual wave

These are orgasms which wax and wane in intensity, but may propagate several times before diminishing. One device sold (the Sybian and similar devices) provides enough continuous stimulation for women to have consistent multiple orgasms. This device has its place in certain specific circumstances which I will mention later.

Orgasm type #8---Multiple orgasms which are staggered

These are orgasms in rhythmic succession. They differ from continual wave orgasms in that they have a more defined resolution and a refractory or recovery state between each orgasm. Each orgasm is specific and individual.

Orgasm type #9---Whole body ---the epitome of orgasms

Whole body orgasms involve a complete momentary catatonic convulsion of the entire body. It is always accompanied by G-spot stimulation of some sort. This is the most elusive of orgasms and I have only witnessed it in five different examples. They are characterized by a catatonic state as the entire body writhes uncontrollably for several seconds. They are also characterized by the woman violently pushing their partner away as they shudder uncontrollably in orgasm and can't stand any further stimulation. They are unmistakable and extremely powerful. If you are lucky enough or skilled enough to attain that level, by all means write an instructional book and spread the information to the rest of us.

Orgasm type #10---Blended/ combination—

A blended orgasm is simply any two or more combined types -this is the most common type of orgasm after clitoral orgasm. The truth is that it is actually difficult to have just a purely clitoral head orgasm because other erogenous areas are tied together. Barring the very light restrictive stimulation precisely on just the clitoral head, it is nearly impossible to not at least trigger some additional response in other areas. Many women have trained themselves to focus on clitoral pleasure and they have partially or completely been unaware of any other erogenous possibilities.

Orgasm type #11---Squirting/ ejaculating—

Both men AND women ejaculate and eject or squirt prostatic fluid at orgasm. There has been quite a disagreement for several years as to whether women actually ejaculate, but the proliferation of recent video and the numerous medical documentations of the content of the fluid have proven that it is a true phenomenon even though it is faked in some sexual encounter scencs. SEXUALLY SKILLED WOMEN EJACULATE SKEIN"S FLUID. The Skene's fluid in female ejaculation varies in viscosity and texture in women, but is pretty similar to the range of ejaculate in men. It seems to be natural for some women and for other women it requires biofeedback response training as I describe elsewhere in this book. SQUIRTING OR EJACULATING ORGASM TRAINING IS AN ABSOLUTELY VITAL PART OF TRAINING FOR WOMEN FOR THEIR ADVANCEMENT OF EASY SEXUAL RESPONSE. Once it becomes a natural response, all other stimulation is markedly enhanced. It is important for all women to open these neural circuits and ejaculate effortlessly.

Orgasm type #12—Oozing as opposed to explosively ejaculating

This is a characteristic of both men and women. Some men and women ejaculate explosively and some ejaculate with a gentle oozing of fluids.

Orgasm type #13---Anal

The stimulation of the anal opening and canal indirectly stimulates all of the rest of the vaginal complex including the G-spot in women and the prostate in men. Obviously careful hygienic practices are absolutely necessary, but many people who have had anal orgasms prefer them to other types.

Orgasm type #14—Skin contraction

A steady temperature increase almost to pain with a water jet on a man's scrotum causes contractions which are a form of orgasmic contractions.

Orgasm type #15—Skin stretching

A gentle rhythmic stretching of the skin with no external skin friction or slippage on a man's penis head and the woman's clitoral hood leads to orgasm. The pleasurable sensation occurs when the skin is gently and rhythmically tensed and released.

Orgasm type #16---Wrapping contraction pressure in men.

This occurs when the vagina is tightened and released rhythmically with no other frictional movement. The stimulation is provided by the woman's vaginal contractions of the PC muscle and the two sets of vertical muscles. More specifics about these muscles will follow in later chapters.

I won't discuss Tantric orgasms here other than to say that it is a particular additional field that you might want to investigate. Until you are somewhat knowledgeable about how to achieve most of the listed types of orgasms, tantric studies might be premature. I do take exception with one premise of Tantric orgasms. PREVENTING the ejaculation of fluids is a primary goal during Tantric sex. In all of my studies and in my experience, it is the expulsion of both male and female sex fluids that bring about some of the most profound sexual and health benefits. The tantric belief is that it is the expulsion of sex fluids that diminishes prana, or life force in your body. I don't believe that.

QUESTIONS and ANSWERS

Here are some interesting questions that seem to come up in many sex study books with some answers included that I hope are useful. They are of general enough interest that I thought it might be useful to at least mention them.

HOW MANY TIMES A WEEK IS IT NORMAL TO HAVE SEX?

It is not unusual for partners in their late teens and twenties to have sex once a day or more. In most couples that tapers down to 3 to 5 times per week as advanced schooling or careers and other activities take attention away from the initial excitement of "all the sex you want" being available. As careers and child rearing take their toll, in the 30 year old to 40 year old group, the typical frequency drops to 2 to 3 times weekly. If the couple is not already bored with each other, that frequency level may continue, but many couples of that age look for alternative interests to the detriment of their sex lives. When menopause sets in at typically about 45 or 50 years old, and the woman is on a hormonal roller coaster or if the man is unable to achieve a hard erection, the couple faces either learning and adapting to changing realities, or avoiding sex altogether. At this stage, it takes pointed effort to keep the sexual interest level high and staleness from entering the bedroom. Those couples who adapt, continue to have a frequency rate that is 2 to 5 times a week with renewed interest and renewed satisfaction which can continue to grow throughout life. If they don't identify the problem and face it, the result is usually a stalemate and often a divorce after the frequency of sex drops to zero. If both partners are committed to each other, their love and sexual expertise can increase as they learn new facts and skills and expand into a very actively and sexually fulfilled state that will last the rest of their lives. Many couples in their 70's and older still have sex twice a week and to some 70's and older couples having sex almost every day. Those are the enlightened couples.

HOW GOOD IS SEX AT DIFFERENT AGES AND HOW DO YOU MEASURE IT?

In the freshness of youth and the adventure of the "forbidden fruit", sex seems easy and natural with raging hormones, a strong heart, toned bodies, and perhaps a hint of rebellion that needs satisfaction. The perfect balance of all of those factors that permit effortless sex become dampened with the inevitable problems of life itself. With making a living, career pressures, advanced educational pressures, having children, or a more complicated social life, the spontaneity can become taxed, sex can morph into a more deliberate planned event if it is even considered at all. At this stage the emphasis may become focused on tried and true techniques because there isn't the desire nor the time to experiment with anything new. "Let's hurry up and get this done!" The sex event becomes only result oriented and not mixed with the joy of trying something new and different. This is the seed of boredom and dissatisfaction and is the precursor to extra marital adventures. Add a feeling of not being appreciated and understood by your mate, female menopausal roller coaster hormone spikes and you are holding a bundle of dynamite with a lit fuse. This is the time that I referred to in the Introduction of this book that I saw so many times in couples when we were running our business.

CAN A SWEET WORD FROM ANYWHERE DURING MENOPAUSE TURN A HEAD AND MAKE YOU OR YOUR MATE DO THINGS YOU WILL REGRET?

You bet it can and does! It can happen any time your mate feels vulnerable.

The boredom stage of dissatisfaction where either or both partners need a sweet word of affection or action from ANY source is when each of us is at our weakest. If a woman really understands the strong restlessness effect menopause has on her, AND her mate does also, together they can minimize the impact the effects of menopause on the psyche of both partners. The helpless feeling women can have of being on a driverless train speeding along at 100 miles an hour with a sharp curve just ahead is a bit more tolerable when she knows that her mate really understands what she is going through. Men, at this point it is not the time to call attention to a bit of tit sagging, a spare tire roll, stretch marks, or a vagina that has done its job of birthing your children and might not be as tight as it once was. Just look into the mirror naked and see if you are still the hot looking stud you were at 19 and cut her some slack. If you can't do that, you are a jackass and you don't deserve her. You might not even recognize that your roving eye is part of your own menopausal dilemma---yes, we men have a form of menopause also, and it is our time of last chances, what ifs, and self-doubt. Whatever you are experiencing, her midlife crisis is probably much worse, and NOW IS THE TIME SHE NEEDS YOUR LOVE AND UNDERSTANDING AND STABILITY THE MOST.

IS IT INEVITABLE FOR BOREDOM TO OCCUR IN A MARRIAGE?

If you both can step back and objectively look at the biological facts at this stage, you have taken the first step toward the renaissance of the most deeply satisfying phase of your sex life that can last through your 80s and beyond. Boredom touches all marriages at some time or another but can be nipped in the bud IF YOR ARE PROACTIVE. Hopefully you both are willing to start having some very frank and open discussions about your own self-image, your life victories and disappointments, and your secret sexual desires and preferences---the ones you were too embarrassed to talk about before. When those subjects are addressed, a new adventure and new excitement will be added in the mix at a time in life when you are more financially secure, the kids are gone and you have the time to use the slightly slower techniques you have hopefully started learning to bring on the big "O" as many times as you desire and do it with complete control and effortless surety as opposed to the hit and miss of using rushed and amateurish techniques.

Oh, to answer the question "How do you measure how good the sex you just had was?" Communicate verbally EXACTLY what is feeling good exactly when it is happening and the answer to that question is automatic. This verbal feedback is a vital part of retraining the erogenous feedback loops as well as the physical signals. Focus on your partner as if they were the ONLY thing in the world at that moment because they should be. Give and you will receive. With that attitude, your sex life will continue to improve. After age 70, it is still improving for my wife and me. I can hardly wait until age 80, or maybe even 90!!! My son's 96 year old Italian father-in-law was seeking instruction from my son about how to access the porn sites on the internet. Go Grandpa!!

IS SEX AN INSTINCT OR DO YOU HAVE TO LEARN HOW TO DO IT?

Actually, any person with absolutely no instruction can instinctively figure out how to put what into what to accomplish fertilization and much pleasure. We seem to instinctively know what goes where and with a little wiggling and jabbing the job gets done. That said, let's compare that level of accomplishment to the concert pianist earlier in the book. If you are content to repeatedly pound out Chop Sticks on the piano and never aspire to Rachmaninoff and Chopin (or even Jerry Lee Lewis) then you will be content to boringly pump away and be a very nominal and predictably boring lover. If you aspire to a multi-faceted sexual repertoire that includes the ability to use several erogenous zones to their maximum level of successful stimulation on demand, then you will have to go to sex-college by studying the previous experiences of those who have gone before you and have devoted much time to their discoveries. This book is a really good start.

I had a conversation one time with a woman when I started writing this book who was puzzled at the idea of anyone who studied sex. She projected an aura as if she already knew all there was to know. Trust me, she didn't know much. She walked away from the conversation with the same ignorance she entered it. I hope this book will induce some questions and provide some answers for people like her. She was so ignorant that she didn't even begin to know what questions to ask.

We are all given a precious and complex instrument for reproduction AND for pleasure and it is a true waste to not learn about our bodies and use them for the greatest health and satisfaction. That includes the therapeutic satisfaction of our partner's psychological and physical being. Sex is, in my opinion, one of the greatest gifts our Creator has given us. In order to properly use it, we have to transcend our inaccurate perceptions about our erogenous zones. Sex does feel good, and is supposed to feel good. There is no guilt here. That is precisely the way God made us---don't forget that. If you learn about your equipment and practice open mindedly and uninhibitedly, you WILL accomplish mastery of your sexual instruments just as the concert pianist masters their Steinway piano and you will transfer that joy to your mate.

WHAT MAKES GOOD SEX? WHAT MAKES BAD SEX?

Quite simply put by the simplest definition, good sex is any sex that feels good and doesn't hurt anyone either physically, or psychologically and bad sex is the opposite.

By another definition, good sex refers to the skill level and good intentions of the participants and bad sex refers to the lack of skill or the employment of bad or manipulative intentions.

Certain people seem to have an innate ability to read a partner and provide the empathy and ability to do or say just the right thing at the right time. They are the "easy studies" that "get it" so that they are already past the communication barrier and can presently begin to learn physical techniques easily. Generally, at least part of their personality is unselfish and they are giving which carries over to the bedroom. The "difficult studies" are those who are selfish and focused on their own pleasure or they are focused on manipulating their partner. They are generally narcissistic. They will need to start by learning to be more focused on others in general and on the needs and desires of their partner in particular. If you are narcissistic, you might start by avoiding the necessity to admire yourself every time you pass by a mirror. Stop concentrating on SELF and focus on others. In the karmic sense, what a person projects is returned with extra added measure. The right intentions are prerequisite for a mastery of a deeply rewarding mutual sex partnership. The study of detailed sexual anatomy and the careful learning of various massaging techniques on specific erogenous spots, timings, and touches is actually a process of simple awareness that all of those things really exist. Then the repeated practice of them over and over is necessary until you can produce orgasms of a specific kind, at will, for your partner. When you can do that, you have earned your proficiency degree in practical sexuality. What I am saying is that the right mental component---the attitude and intent is actually even more important than the physical component— DON"T FORGET THIS. It goes in this sequence----

> correct attitude first and foremost
> shedding of inhibitions
> a loving and experimental mindset
> mastery physical stimulation skills

If any of those components is out of order or aren't present, things just will not work right. Techniques are developed over weeks, months and even years and trying to rush it will result in frustration. Patience, patience, patience with yourself and with your partner leads to success. Impatience leads to failure.

WHAT IS SEXUAL IMPRINTING? ---- (IMPORTANT)

We are all imprinted sexually and it is deeply rooted and is the single most powerful influence on our inhibitions, our attitudes and the success of our sex lives.

We become the exact sexual combination of open mindedness or inhibition starting with our earliest memories. From the first word of admiration or the first word of ridicule from our crib to the grade school playground, we start forming our self-image. As we interact with parents, with friends, strangers and even with the mirror, we are constantly forming or reinforcing our feelings of self-worth and confidence OR we are tearing down our self-image. How easy it is to react to an unkind or thoughtless remark in a negative way that plants itself into our memories. It gets stuck in our subconscious to be raked up and be mentally replayed and magnified each time we hear some thoughtless remark directed toward us. The negatives magnify over time if we don't have a balanced opinion of ourselves. This is true of all words, but is especially true of ANYTHING remotely relating to physical or sexual desirability. Lowered self-esteem and magnified inhibitions is the result. The world is full of examples of low self-esteem individuals (both men and women) who have been targeted by manipulative and predatory individuals who use any person with a lower self-esteem as a kicking dog. Somehow they feel a sense of power in the reduction of another person to buoy themselves up. I make this point because a healthy self-esteem is vital to a fulfilled sexual relationship. OUR FIRST SEXUAL EXPERIENCE IS A FILTER THROUGH WHICH ALL OF OUR SUBSEQUENT EXPERIENCES ARE SUBCONSCIOUSLY COMPARED. Read that sentence over several times. If a particular song was playing, that will always be associated with the experience---good or bad. The exact location such as the seat of a car, the floor, or a bed, the exact timing of technique, type of technique, presence or lack of orgasm, whether the lights were on or off, a particular sexual sound, or a smell, or even a barking dog all imprint on us. All of those seemingly insignificant things will forever be associated with our first sexual experience. Even whether our first experience was riddled with guilt, a tender or a rough partner, or ANYTHING associated with the experience itself and a full compilation of our self-image at the time sets the stage for how we will likely function for DECADES to come by triggering associated memories of the event. Most of us tend to magnify any positive or negative input we perceive. If our self-esteem is on the negative side, the input will tend to be perceived to the negative, and if the individual has a positive self-esteem, the input will tend be perceived to the positive. Just a smile from a tall, dark, and handsome man can be a momentous experience for a woman with low self-esteem, but positive comments might even be expected by a woman with a robust self-esteem and even go unnoticed because she is so used to continually hear positive comments. The healthy balance is somewhere between self-loathing and conceit. Sort of the "I'm O.K., you're O.K." balance of healthy self-acceptance.

PAY PARTICULAR ATTENTION TO THE NEXT TWO PARAGRAPHS. THEY MAY BE THE MOST IMPORTANT PARAGRAPHS IN THIS BOOK.

This is a repeat and a more detailed enforcement of something I said earlier. There are nerve circuits attached to all erogenous zones that respond to the memory of smells, sounds, touches, flashes of a visions, and even fantasized ideas. These circuits will go dormant if they are not exercised and if they are never awakened early in life, they will need to be coaxed into service by an understanding partner and a willing subject who has dropped at least some of their own inhibitions. All inhibitions are challenges to be conquered if you are to achieve a really robust sex life.

Unless you are already aware of, and are proficient in stimulating all of the erogenous zones listed in chapter VII, YOU HAVE DORMANT CIRCUITS THAT NEED AWAKENING.

The first step is understanding that these circuits exist but that they are very likely closed down by inhibitions. I have had years of personal experience in this area and I assure you it is real. The impact of dealing with it is probably the most important thing I have discovered regarding sex. It has to be addressed one specific erogenous zone at a time with a combination of discussions and actual stimulating practice with real time very detailed uninhibited feedback from the partner. With the right dedication and love, any circuit that has been dormant can be awakened. Once it is awakened, it remains functional. Once you are able to open at least one of the four "G"-spot circuits to allow for true female ejaculation (see Chapter VIII on techniques) the other circuits will follow with much less effort.

IS IT NORMAL TO MASTURBATE?

In a word, YES, it is completely normal! Masturbation as the normal way young adolescents learn about at least some of their body function. In most studies published by sex researchers, masturbation is shown to be normal and even desirable behavior except in a few rare and extreme pathologic cases. The frequency generally ranges from daily to occasionally. The combined statistics show that those individuals who started masturbating as youngsters had a better sexual understanding, better sexual function, and less inhibitions than those who hadn't. Many more people have practiced masturbation than haven't. The reasons range all over the map. It is used to release sexual hormone buildup and stress relief in all ages and both sexes. It is practiced just because it feels good, and as a substitute for sex when the partner isn't available. It is practiced by men who want to dramatically reduce their risk of prostate cancer or to open the prostate as the hormones pass by and temporarily relax the constriction of an enlarged prostate. Masturbation is a practice that most often is part of a person's sex life for their entire life. All of the recently available vibrators and dildos for women and vaginal reproductions of cyberskin for men have made masturbation easier and more realistic options for any number of situations. Tens of millions of masturbation aids are sold worldwide each year and that alone attests to their widespread use in addition to the old tried and true natural hand method. It is not uncommon for women to even carry some form of miniature vibrator in their purse for handy use.

James A. Grant

HOW DO SEXUAL PRACTICES DIFFER
AMONG DIFFERENT CULTURES?

We tend to perceive our attitudes of sex in the United States as somewhat decadent because of the wide use of sex in advertising and in all media. Actually, the opposite is true. In the modern cultures of the West, we publicly have one of the most prudish attitudes of sex in the world, but not privately. In other words, our society is hypocritical on the subject.

Without doing an anthropological study on numerous cultures, suffice it to say that sexual practices and "norms" wary widely.

As the sailors and explorers of the sixteenth, seventeenth and eighteenth century found out, most native cultures of the New World, the South Seas, and Africa had sexual rituals and practices that included everything from parents deflowering their own children to "break them in" and also to educate them, sharing wives with guests, fertility orgies, and open communal sex sharing. Orgies have been with mankind throughout history predating Greek times, through Roman times, and all the way through Ben Franklin and up to present times. Open and less inhibited sexual practices were generally somewhat more common to the higher political or financial echelons. We just aren't told much about it in the history books. Concubines were common in the Old Testament, temple prostitutes were an accepted part of some societies, pluralistic marriages common in the Mormon Church until laws were passed against it by outsiders in the late nineteenth century, and a small percentage of about 4% the population is presently active in formal swinger enclaves all over the world. We have been guided in our perceptions of reality in modern America by those who want to control us.

Just as the sex researchers have shown over and over, what we thought was reality didn't match what people actually did.

WHAT SEX POSITION IS BEST?

Some of this section on positions is necessarily detailed and is pretty graphic, but it would not really be useful unless it was so explicit. After all, we are all adults here.

Compiled by Vatsyayana in a text taken from a previous Hindu text dating from 200 to 400 A.D, the Kama Sutra depicts at least sixty four sex positions. The compiled text was translated and brought to Western Europe in 1883 by Sir Richard Burton (not the actor who married Elizabeth Taylor). It created quite a stir at the time. I have seen further text versions showing nearer 100 different positions. To this Westerner, most of them seem very impractical and frankly don't ring my bell and that may just exemplify how much I still have to learn. A few positions are very practical and very efficient for aiding the stimulation of the very specific orgasmic targets mostly directed toward the female's orgasm. If you are highly experimental and you are athletic, by all means, try them all. I have concentrated on the ones which do a very specific thing. They get results for me. Your best bet is to sit down with a copy of the illustrated versions and talk it over with your partner and decide how gymnastic you want to be. Although many of the positions are fun to try and are interesting, I have found that only a half dozen or so positions produce the biggest bang for the buck (pun intended). If you are already 70, don't get too adventurous here or you might end up with a broken something in your gymnastic contortions.

MISSIONARY POSITION

The missionary position allows a diversity of angular penetration that can stimulate the clitoris, the G-spot, the U-spot, the cervix, and the A-spot. Just a slight tilt of the female's hips directs the thrust directly toward the correct target, allowing her the precise control at all times. Her mastery of the positioning of her pubic bone by tucking her hips upward and forward (scooping) will determine the specific angle of penetration and thereby the exact point of stimulation. Most women don't inherently have a clue as to the places they should be targeting unless they are first aware of their specific erogenous zones and practice stimulation exercises together with continuous verbal feedback from her partner so she can picture in her mind what is happening inside her vagina. Men can see their penis as they explore it, but women need to be told "I am touching your cervix, you're A- spot, your U-spot, etc." and, "does this circular motion feel better or do you like this come hither motion better?" Women don't have a sense of their geography because they can't see inside themselves and it is difficult for them to mentally isolate the stimulation at first until they make the necessary associations with verbal feedback going both ways. It is next to impossible for a woman to efficiently explore all of these zones without a dedicated partner to experiment with and communicate with. Men, that is your job and I assure you that it is an embarkation of a journey that will fascinate and reward you. Most men and women default to the clitoris because it is the most prominent part and the easiest to find. Most women know something about their clitoris because they have played with it, but without the help of a partner, her hope to understand the rest of her equipment alone is pretty restricted. After several to many of these sessions, all of the benefits of the various angles of penetration and positions become pretty automatic.

In the missionary position, if the woman draws up her legs with them wide open, the pelvic bone is most exposed and allows for the deepest penetration of the vagina which tugs at all other parts including the clitoral root, it will produce an A-spot orgasm if the man is long enough or is using a long dildo. Just a few correctly timed and targeted thrusts in this position can cause deep satisfying orgasms for the woman. The man penetrates as deep as possible with very firm pressure just the correct angle with the woman NOT using the pubic bone as a fulcrum (allowing deep direct firm stretching of the full vaginal length). Well-endowed men need to be very careful in this position and not exceed the comfort zone of the woman. The woman can sharply increase both partners' sensations by drawing up her knees while simultaneously rocking and tilting her hips and legs rhythmically (scooping) while she is in the missionary position. Not enough women know this technique. It is VERY important! A variation that is also very effective is for the woman to "leg lock" around her partners waist or thighs and draw herself forcefully against him with her heels while bumping and grinding her clitoris against his pubic bone.

COWGIRL AND REVERSE COWGIRL POSITION

The "cowgirl" position (female on top face to face) allows extreme clitoral stimulation, "U" spot stimulation, and full control by the female. It used to be called the "French" position when I was young. The female squats over the man with her knees on either side of him. Because of gravity, the internal female parts are pressed downward and outward and are positioned for more friction. Many women consider this their favorite position. Reverse "cowgirl" is the same female riding on top position with the woman turned around facing towards her prone partner's feet. By scooping forward and rocking her hips forward and back (either with the knees on or off the bed), using her pubic bone as a fulcrum, she can make her movements massage all deeper internal G-spot, cervical, and A-spot zones. The more the female rocks her hips forward and back in a scooping motion, the more control and stimulation she will have and the more stimulation she will give to her partner. Many of the most intense female orgasms result from using these cowgirl positions. If I was to pick out the single physical action that improves sexual performance, it is THE MASTERY BY THE WOMAN OF HER HIP SCOOPING ACTION. That is true of all positions. In numerous observations, it is evident to me that the more a woman scoops her hips, the more accomplished her sexual skill and prowess.

One of the most highly skilled and completely uninhibited mature aged women I have ever viewed in a sex session used the cowgirl position to scoop her hips. She stimulated her G-spot by scooping with an inserted penis, then scooped her opened vaginal lips and clitoris against the underside of her husband's penis a few times and switched back to internal stimulation and a G-spot orgasm, squirted and then inserted his penis inside again and only one firm deep thrust triggered her A- spot to an instant second orgasm simultaneously with her husband. Very effective.

The face sitting cowgirl position with the female on top straddling her partner's head is also a popular cunnilingus position because it allows the man the full access of the deepest possible areas including the #1 G-spot, a partial access to the #2 G-spot as gravity drops the G-spot area closer to the entrance of the vagina, the U-spot and the clitoris, and the inner labia. This position, even without any direct stimulation to the man is very erotic just from the smells of the female hormones and pheromones which mist the area.

DOGGIE POSITION

The "doggie" is just like the name implies---the man enters the vagina from behind with the woman on all fours just like canines do it. Again, most women don't understand the complexity of their anatomy and just view their vagina as a hole, but it is infinitely more complex and wonderful than that. The thing she has to remember is that SHE has the aiming apparatus and controls the precise internal target by using her pubic bone and her hip angle and motion to direct the penetration precisely where SHE wants it. ALL WOMEN NEED TO KNOW THIS AND USE THIS FORM OF CONTROL, particularly if her partner has limited skills himself and doesn't know how to aim for the right spots. The missionary position only stimulates the clitoris indirectly by tugging the clitoral root, so it is a good position to locate the A-spot, the cervix, and the two innermost positions of the G-spot. The man can get particular pleasure in this position because his frenulum (it is the cleft on underside of the penis head) rubs the hard ring of the cervix if the woman knows what she is doing, she can "re-sight" her vagina with slight hip tilts to target the exact area she wants to stimulate and change momentarily the stimulus to favor herself and then her partner and have full control of the timing of the orgasm for herself and of for her partner.

THE "69" POSITION

In addition to the above positions for intercourse, the old "69" oral position with the woman on top is a favorite for many couples. It allows the most freedom with the most diverse oral options of stimulation, and with the full enjoyment of the options of the man smelling and tasting the wonderful female fluids and smelling the hormonal musk. It allows the woman the most flexibility to do whatever she wants. Some couples consider this to be the most personal and encompassing of all sexual contact.

MALE STANDING POSITION

Another extremely effective position for direction of the penis to the exact right target is the "male standing position", where the woman is on her back extending her legs over the edge of the bed with legs either drawn up to her chest or bent down to the floor with the man standing on the floor. Most beds are close enough to the right height to allow for the correct coupling position. Additional pillows are sometimes useful when placed under the woman's hips. It allows a restful, but very effective slow rhythmic and very controlled motion at .8 Hertz while allowing the woman complete control over angle of penetration. A variation is the man on the floor on his knees (on a pillow) with the woman on the edge of the bed with knees drawn up for a very comfortable cunnilingus.

In my personal and observational experience, the above positions are the most productive and I'm sure that there are many others that you might wish to explore, but I have chosen to spend my emphasis exploring the sexual stimulating motions for the maximum rewards. You might disagree after trying others.

AGAIN, RESTATING A VITAL POINT, ALL WOMEN NEED TO KNOW AND PRACTICE THE TILTING AND AIMING (HIP SCOOPING) TECHNIQUE IN ALL POSITIONS.

The vast majority of women haven't learned to use their pubic bone correctly, just as the vast number of men aren't aware of the precise locations of all the major erogenous areas that women possess. In such cases, they are both shooting in the dark and any successes are accidental.

IS IT NORMAL TO ENGAGE IN ORAL SEX?

It is a prevailing and common practice to engage in fellatio and cunnilingus either individually alternatively or simultaneously. If a person was raised in a restrictive environment, the practice may seem crude and even disgusting. It is my opinion that a person should only do what they want to do, but I would certainly not eliminate it before trying it at least a few times. If you choose to not engage in oral sex, you will be eliminating a large portion of very satisfying experiences from your life. Cleanliness is important, but remember that the natural secretions of both men and women are biological triggers. A sanitary and clean body frames the pleasantry of the other "fresh" genital scents. Raunchy is raunchy. The difference between powerful natural musky pheromones and just plain raunchy isn't difficult to discern. Excess use of perfumes and colognes disguise the natural pheromones that are so potent to natural sexual attraction and stimulation.

IS THERE SUCH A THING AS A BAD ORGASM?

Orgasms differ greatly in duration, intensity, and in the "shape" of their personality. Some orgasms are just a quiet bump, and some are absolutely mind blowing and encompass quaking tremors that rock the entire body. An old high school girlfriend of mine whom I hadn't seen for over 50 years recently said something out of the blue one day which I chuckled at and fully agreed with. She said "There is no such thing as a bad orgasm!!" (I will point out that she had been married to a devoted husband for about 49 years at the time she said that, and her comment had come from her own personal married experience). That pretty much sums it up about orgasms. Acquiring the many skills to achieve the best kind of each type of orgasm is not only possible, but necessary to have a really fulfilled sex life with all of its physical and psychological benefits. The wonderful thing is that with self-training, age doesn't matter and your best orgasms are still in your future if you are willing to become more informed and are willing to practice. The life balancing release of a really intense orgasm is one of the high points of life that should be regularly repeated. I love flying small airplanes and orgasms are right up there with the mental intensity and emotion of landing an airplane in a severe storm with a maximum crosswind. It really gets your full attention! Learning to repeat good orgasms regularly is a wonderful skill. My wife was a French student and she says the French have an appropriate saying for it----"La Petite Mort"! In English it roughly translates to "the little death"!

IS IT NORMAL TO ENGAGE IN ANAL SEX?

Anal sex is a widely controversial subject. Some cultures consider it completely normal and some consider it absolutely taboo. In some societies it is illegal. It is very widely practiced all over the world in secret and due to the very personal sensitive nature of it, the subject is almost never brought up in polite society. In addition to being a significant practice in the heterosexual community, it is the prime emphasis in the male gay community. It is also practiced in the lesbian community using dildos or finger stimulation. Anal orgasms can be some of the most intense orgasms one can experience, particularly when they involve the anterior anal ridge. Careful attention to ultra-cleanliness is obviously important to prevent infections, and great care must be exercised to prevent injuries because of the delicacy of anal tissue. Paraphrasing the conversation of Dr. Ruth again, a guest sexologist as a guest on a late night talk show stated that, as a sexologist, she approved of anal sex, but that no vaginal or oral entry should be done in the session after anal penetration has occurred. If anal sex is a moral issue for you, then do only what you think is proper for you.

IS IT NORMAL TO HAVE MULTIPLE SEX PARTNERS?

This is actually two questions. If you are speaking about threesomes, foursomes, etc., and orgies, the answer is that a small percentage of the population practices those regularly. I haven't read any study that attributed any more than 4% of the population that practice them. Taking the projected percentage of 4%, in a town of 10,000 population, then 400 of those 10,000 people would practice threesomes, foursomes, and orgies on a regular basis. It is likely that some people on your block are some of them. I suspect that a higher percentage than 4% might have tried it once or twice, but not regularly.

If you are talking about one person having a variety of sex partners over time, the percentage is much higher, particularly among unattached adults. The encounters can be casual one night stands or affairs that last weeks, months or years. There are such things as "open" marriages where both partners condone sexual relations with others, usually with some sort of ground rules. They consider sex much the same as a nice meal to be enjoyed with no recriminations or guilt and the participants don't attach an emotional consideration to their affairs. The couples who practice open marriages have to be very secure in their relationship for it to work. Sometimes the word polyamory is used to describe those people who truly love more than one mate or other person. Others consider their marriages a business contract and extramarital sex is allowed and expected, and the rest of the marriage stays intact for business reasons, cultural reasons, or family continuity. Many rich and famous families operate in this realm. In these arrangements, being discrete is usually the sacred rule. It might also be interesting to note that many of the people who condone this kind of relationships are also regular attendees of church services (probably also for appearances sake).

IS FANTASIZING NORMAL DURING SEX?

I have read several studies on this subject and they all seem to be pretty universal in their conclusion that fanaticizing during sex is very common and completely natural so if you do it, don't beat yourself up. Fantasies can include almost anything. The most common fantasy is sex with other people than your mate, group sex, forbidden sex of any sort, sex with a previous partner, sex with a prostitute or gigolo, giving sex for money, forced sex, fetishes, pain, sadism and masochism, watching your mate have sex with someone else, sex with strangers, sex with neighbors, sex in public, sex with an authority figure, sex with a movie star or a favorite singer, and sex with the danger of being caught in the act by your mate. The list is almost endless. The consensus among sex researchers is that these fantasies are harmless, normal, and are a healthy way to spice up your sex life. One survey which is pretty typical stated that 71 % of men regularly fantasize, and

72% of women regularly fantasize. It seems to be pretty equal across genders. Some subjects have reported that their fantasies are a prerequisite for them to come to orgasm which at that point makes them a fetish for those individuals. Sexual fantasies are likely to secretly be even more prevalent in long term marriages.

IS ROLL PLAY NORMAL DURING SEX?

Roll play is the extension of fantasizing in which both partners join in a story scenario and act out the characters and even include props and special clothing. It is also a very normal practice. People who enjoy a high degree of sexual freedom in their thinking and a low level of inhibitions find the practice of roll play very exhilarating and a good way to add variety and spice to their sexual repertoire. If you are able to roll play comfortably, you are a really good candidate to employ all of the information in this book to enhance your skills because you already are cooperating and communicating as a couple and the other learning steps will be natural and fun to you. If you can't bring yourself to either roll play or at least fantasize, you are probably pretty inhibited and need to loosen up and take yourself less seriously.

CHAPTER VIII

DETAILED SPECIFIC TECHNIQUES

Any discussion on specific techniques needs to be prefaced by stressing once again that INHIBITIONS ARE THE KILLER TO A GOOD SEX LIFE because inhibitions are the cause of repression of the feedback loops of erotic stimulation. Please RE-READ THAT SENTENCE until it is planted firmly in your recall.

If you are 20 years old or 80 years old, your sexual stimulation circuits must be DISCOVERED and ACTIVATED by repetitive and directed stimulation including both the body and the mind. An 80 year old might have gone through her entire life with only the one circuit to the clitoral head being discovered and activated. What about the clitoral root, the U-spot, the G-spot, the A-spot, the nipple circuit and all of the other circuits discussed in previously in CHAPTER VII. Since the clitoral head is external and easy to find, many women never get past developing the feedback circuits for all of the other erogenous areas that are not externally visible and are harder to locate and thereby are harder to train. Since they have found that the clitoral head gets the job done, they take the lazy route and that becomes the pinnacle of their sexual understanding. That's like only playing two keys on a grand piano and never knowing what all of the other keys or knowing what the pedals do. That leads to pretty boring music. The fact that so few people know anything about some of the other erogenous circuits, and the continued uncertainty even in sex researcher's texts and medical texts is shocking testament that the information needs to be passed on in a specific and detailed manner.

Using that as a starting point, and assuming that you are a patient person and you are committed to sexual improvement, let's get on with the description of specific techniques that will open the circuits to discovering and awakening all of your sexual assets. Remember that I make no claim about being an expert. I am just a devoted practitioner of sex with a lot of patience and with a curious mind that has studied and practiced what I have included in this book. I hope that others might find my collection of information and experience to be valuable.

Since this book is entitled "SEX AFTER SEVENTY", one thing I will discuss is the use of dildos, because over half of men after 50 have some form of erectile dysfunction. Don't worry, some of the best orgasms for women are produced with a dildo rather than a live penis. Younger couples also need to do a significant part of their training using dildos because many things are easier to discover and to control using them. Men, don't get insecure on me here because you likely will find that being at the helm of a really good cyberskin dildo with a modified handle gives you more control and endurance and effectiveness than you ever had with your precious hard penis. What's really exciting is that you have a front row seat to watch every detail of what that wonderful vagina is doing all throughout the session. You will be amazed at what you learn, and you will have the love of your life singing happy songs. She will love you more each time for your efforts. Before you can completely understand the effective use of dildos, you'll need to learn VAGINAL GEOGRAPHY.

VAGINAL GEOGRAPHY

I call this section vaginal geography rather than vaginal physiology because this book is about sexual skill rather than naming exact functions and parts by their scientific names and describing their actual scientific functions. Sexual physiology is an interesting study to pursue if you want more specifics in more scientific terms, but my guess is that you are probably more interested in direct and practical information in layman's terms. You can find anything you want to research on the internet, but be prepared for the inevitable conflicting information between sites and reports. That part can be pretty frustrating. I will only reference the several parts that I know and love. I suspect there are more yet to be discovered by the medical experts, but that is another matter.

I repeat that a vagina is not just a hole, or a collapsed tube. That was the most shocking thing I learned when I had my first real sexual experience. It is not exactly tubular and it is not at all simple. It took me a long time to fully appreciate that it is a very complex instrument made up of several very different triggers, switches and textures, and the textures constantly change throughout the sex act. It has the great feature of secreting a cocktail of lubricants and hormones. The texture of the inside of a human vagina can be smooth like the surface of a balloon, it can be ridged with various patterns resembling very coarse fingerprints in certain areas, or it can be roughly textured throughout with a surface which is more like the top of the tongue, it may also have many light to heavy folds, or may be more coarsely rough. Most men have never really seen inside vaginas the way a gynecologist would and are probably so horny as soon as they get down there that they go for the easy thrill by just stimulating the woman's clitoris----- big mistake. This is probably where all of your years of experience have let you down because if you are like most men and women, you didn't realize there was so much to know about the female vagina. Women can't know everything about their own vagina because without their mate's help, THEY CAN'T SEE ALL OF IT even if they try.

WHETHER YOU ARE A 30 YEAR OLD OR 60 YEARS OLD, THIS WILL BE NEW TERRITORY

Since the vagina is positioned so that even with mirrors, women never really get a good look at it, they can't accurately relate any sensations they have by inserting anything into it themselves. This is where an enlightened partner has to do the exploring and verbally relay the information to them as the partner discovers all of the mysteries. Then both partners are able to relay information back and forth so that she can identify all of the new sensations with the particular movements that her partner is making and describing. She slowly learns to mentally equate specific sensations to the sleeping locations she wasn't aware of. It becomes an exercise in bio-feedback. The male partner using a dildo and fingers is the best way this can be done. Your penis is almost useless here. The penis doesn't have the tactility nor the flexibility and mobility of either fingers or a dildo. Men---- stop thinking "penis"! Exact techniques on this will follow under the heading ---SQUIRTING (FEMALE EJACULATION).

Gynecologists observe many different types of vaginas, but their field is birthing babies and determination of health and of possible unhealthy pathology. Actual sexual pleasure knowledge isn't the primary role for the gynecologist. Any gynecological studies that I have read seem to show an indifference or a lack of knowledge about actual advanced vaginal sexual response. In their defense, by law and by ethics, they can't be involved with the sexual stimulation of a patient during a gynecological examination. It is difficult to believe that the debate is still being bantered about that there is no such thing as a vaginal orgasm and that female ejaculate is only urine! We are way beyond that.

VAGINAS ARE REALLY DIVERSE

Adding to the information in the previous chapter about the physical map of a vagina, there are even more characteristics and differences. Vaginas differ greatly in diameter, length, and texture from person to person and each one of those things effects the sexual feeling to that particular woman and to her partner. The particular size, internal texture, and muscular pelvic strength will determine any particular woman's sexual response and also will determine the specific degree of sexual response for her partner with any given motion. The only way to know anything about your particular woman is to examine her vagina with a speculum and a flashlight. Surgical stainless speculums are available for $15 on E-bay. Go VERY slowly, be EXTREMELY gentle and use plenty of water based lubricant such as KY jelly when you do this. Make note of exactly what you see and describe it to her. Feel just behind the pubic bone and locate the transverse ridges of the G spot on the front side (anterior) of the vagina behind the pubic bone. The #3 G-spot is a gristly and roughly textured bump about the size of an unshelled almond. Note its texture. It changes constantly during stimulation. At times it flattens down and almost disappears, at times it is very rough feeling and at times it is engorged with Skenes fluid and feels puffy. Feel for every bump and hollow in front and back of it and note the underlying gristly ureter passage by using firm finger pressure against the inside of the pubic bone. Hard side to side stimulation pressure is very sensual to the woman. You will feel the ureter passage slip back and forth under your finger. There are 4 separate areas in front of, on, and in back of the transverse ridges that will create 4 distinct orgasms. If it is possible, carefully feel the donut shaped cervix which is a couple inches above and behind the transverse ridges of the G-spot. Note its shape and texture. You won't be able to visually observe the A-spot at the upper end of the vagina without a speculum and it is difficult to discern anyway because it doesn't have a distinctive structure. Practice different pressures, timings, come hither motion and circular motion with fingers on all areas from the cervix outward to the urethra (pee hole) and on up to the outside of the vagina and up to the clitoral hood and head. Note the difference in sensitivity of the clitoris through the hood and also without the hood and note the difference of sensitivity when the vaginal lips are gently spread open and the clitoris head is fully exposed AND in mild tension by VERY GENTLY stretching the skin sideways with two fingers away from the clitoral head. Always be sure to use plenty of water based lubrication unless you are using your tongue. Remember that the surface of the clitoris head is as sensitive as an eyeball because it has more nerve endings than anywhere else in the body. Also remember that according to several sources, it has over twice the number of nerve endings as the male penis head and is many times smaller, so the nerves are even more concentrated in such a small area so it is much more sensitive than your penis head. When she says "MMMM" at any point and shows her pleasure, PAY ATTENTION, make note of it, and TELL HER EXACTLY what you are doing as you do it. She doesn't know and can't tell what you are doing unless you tell her. She must learn to make the mental associations and only you can communicate that to her. To her it seems like a general sensation in a general area until she can assign a feeling to a specific location repeatedly. She just knows that it is feeling good. It is normal for a woman to want very firm pressure at times and extremely gentle and light pressure at other times. It is up to you to be responsive to her changing desires by being observant of sounds and micro movements. Go with her desires and learn to develop the sixth sense of reading her responses and micro movements. Next, focus away from the clitoris. Focus again on the anterior or frontal wall of the inside of the vagina. Pay particular attention to the delicate hollows. Press against her pubococcygeal muscle (PC muscle) about an inch inside her vaginal opening and feel how it attaches to the pubic bone and note what happens when she flexes it. Give her EXACTLY what she wants for stimulation and not what you want. Also note how slight differences in her reaction to pressure sideways rolling the finger left to right, or come hither front to back with either one finger or with a walking two fingered motion on the G-spot area. Press outward on all areas of her PC muscle to give her a sense of dimension. Make precise mental notes of her exact response on any area. You are just now getting acquainted with her vagina and you are actually mapping her individual personal responses. Used properly at a slow rate of .8 Hertz, your fingerprint ridges are very erotic to her. Be aware of it. If you give in to the natural tendency to do everything too fast, her ability to respond will diminish because the sensations are more muted. She should be talking to you about EXACTLY what she is experiencing and you should continually be doing the same for her. You are in the process of bonding on a psychological level you likely never experienced before because you are intimate and verbally communicating with focused attention only on each other. Keep these sessions up until they are as normal as talking about the weather. Use them as foreplay or use them all the way to orgasm. Don't have a rigid agenda. If she finishes any session with a pleasant experience, you both have won and you become bonded more closely. More importantly, you will reinforce her mental picture about what it feels like to her when you do a particular thing and her all-important mental association for the reactive imprinting will begin to be activated and it will become automatic in her active mental imaging in future sessions. This is true for ANY stimulation.

CLITORAL DIFFERENCES AMONG WOMEN

The size, exact position of the clitoris, the prominence of a clitoral hood, the absence or presence of an external clitoral shaft, or the length of a clitoral shaft if it is present all have some bearing on the particular ease with which a woman can have a clitoral orgasm and whether her clitoris is directly stimulated in particular intercourse positions. Some clitoral shafts are barely visible bumps and some are vertically erectile like a small penis. There shouldn't be too much made of the differences, because all clitorises are highly sensitive. At least a mention should be made of the differences because the position, size and structure of the clitoris has some bearing on the ease of stimulation.

Just as approximately 95% of men have penises that are considered average size with only about 5% having significantly larger ones, a similar percentage of female clitoris heads are somewhere around the same average size when compared to each other. I haven't seen any studies directly related to this in females, so this hypothesis is only the result of pictorial study. Only a small percentage of clitoris heads are significantly larger than the size of two pencil eraser ends. A small percentage of women have clitoral heads as large as a thumbnail and with an erectile shaft that acts very much like a miniature erect penis which is 1 to 2 inches long. Very rarely, a clitoral shaft is over 3 inches long. It appears that some women body builders have large clitorises and clitoral shafts perhaps from taking male hormones to help them bulk up.

The size of the clitoral hood which covers the clitoral head is significant in the ease of access to direct stimulation, but a large or very fleshy clitoral hood is certainly not a deal breaker. It just means that the hood has to be gently pulled back to expose the head to direct stimulation when that is the specific stimulation she wants. Many women actually prefer the main stimulation to be slightly above the clitoral head. Either partner can perform the necessary action of spreading and holding the vaginal lips open to expose the clitoral head from behind the sheath when it is desired. It is just something that both partners should be aware of.

One European study concluded that the distance between the clitoral head and the G-spot had a bearing on the ease with which woman can have a G-spot orgasm. I'm no scientist, but I would like to see more study on this before I venture an opinion. I'm not presently convinced about that.

In some positions of intercourse (particularly the missionary position), a long clitoral shaft could be a distinct advantage for the woman to receive the most direct contact.

PENIS SHAPES, SIZES, AND PERSONALITIES--- FROM WOMEN'S POINT OF VIEW---DOES SIZE MATTER?

Since the male penis is so prominent and attached on the exterior of the body, it is out in the open for easy observation and it has few secrets. There isn't a universal classification of human male penises that I have found anywhere, so I will use my own system of classification and description. I have listened to and watched several interviews of all ages of women ranging in age from late teens to elderly women about the eternal question of "Does size matter?" They also tell their individual preferences about what shape, size and personality of penis they prefer. The women generally interviewed had experienced numerous different sexual partners and that particular knowledge would only be available from someone with that specific experience. I think after consideration that their opinions are relevant and informative and valuable to pass on because the methods of almost all of the several surveys I have viewed were non-sensational, matter-of-fact, and the answers appeared to have the ring of truth and sincerity to me. They seemed also to be pretty similar from study to study. You decide for yourself.

The different surveys had a wide range of focus, but the common elements are reported here. There is no distinct relationship of the size of a flaccid penis and the same penis after erection. Some penises just expand more than others as they become erect.

Male human penises as measured erect (measured firmly against the pubic bone on the top side of the penis to the end), vary in size from approximately 2 inches to as long as 11 inches with the average being about 5 to 6 inches for the North American male. That average figure varies slightly from study to study. There are rumored reports of a very few which are up to 13 ½ inches in length. Very few men are anywhere close to either the shortest or longest extreme. The several surveys on the subject of size don't exactly agree, but they are all pretty close as far as AVERAGE typical length goes. The legendary debate of the effectiveness of an extra-long penis as a tool of sexual satisfaction is greatly exaggerated in the opinion of many women. Some women disagree and prefer men with long penises. The length is only one component of size. Diameter and girth are the other significant dimensions. Some very long penises are not large in girth, and some short penises are large in girth. As you read further chapters, imagine how all of these differences might affect stimulation of the U-spot, the G-spot, the A-spot and the cervix as well as what the friction would be inside a vagina which is extremely elastic and adapts to most sizes automatically. The vagina is extremely accommodating to different sizes and shapes of penises. Whether a penis is exactly straight, curved up, curved down, or curved sideways is a factor for sex in certain positions. Other factors are whether it is exactly round in cross section or somewhat flattened or oval in cross section. Whether the head is a much greater diameter than the shaft, or whether the shaft diameter is about the same as the head are other important factors as to exactly how a particular size and shape will be effective as it is used in different techniques.

I list some of the general different types according to my own somewhat arbitrary classification because I can't find a system of classification in general use. I will also mention their strong and weak points, and also the personalities that many women have assigned to men with differing types of penises. It should be no surprise that a man's penis size would tend to effect his self-image and his personality much the same as breast sizes and shapes effect women.

SOME PENIS TYPES, ADVANTAGES AND DISADVANTAGES

A section shortly follows to further explain the techniques of using the various types of penises or with dildos to hit a woman's erogenous spots under the heading—"LEARN THE BASICS WITH ENTHUSIASM—HERE THEY ARE".

LANCE

This a fairly straight and uniform penis of any length. It has a head that is slightly larger than the shaft. The longer ones are great for hitting the A-spot, the mid sizes and shorter ones are the all-purpose tools that are average for everything else. Women generalize that guys with long lances have a high opinion of themselves because they have high level bragging rights among men. The disadvantage is that if they are too long, they prevent the man from bumping directly against the woman's pubic bone and clitoris which many women say that they like. If they are not used gently, the lance can be uncomfortable and hurt the woman with too much pressure against the upper end of her vagina.

MUSHROOM

This type is distinctive because the head is abruptly much larger than the shaft. It can be any length and is particularly effective for hitting the G-spot, the U-spot, and the cervix. The larger diameter head is pleasant for many women surveyed because they like the friction of the abrupt shaped head with a slight restriction at the PC muscle due to the large head. Most mushrooms are average length, so it is difficult to stimulate the A-spot with them.

BANANA

This type curves up and is particularly shaped for easily stimulating all G-spot areas and the cervix. Most bananas are average size and if the woman is lazy or ignorant about scooping her hips correctly, the banana shape which curves up allows things to sort of work even without any female hip movement. Bananas work well for inexperienced women that don't understand the importance of moving and tilting their hips. Most women like bananas as an overall multi-purpose shape. The banana gives the impression of a more youthful erection since it looks perky. Since bananas are not usually especially long, they aren't particularly superior to stimulate the A-spot but are good for everything else.

STUBBY

These are larger than average diameter and tend to be a little bit shorter than average. Their distinction is that the shaft is unusually thick, but not particularly long and the head is just slightly larger than the shaft. Many women actually like the stubby and it probably has something to do with the length of their individual vaginas. Several women complained about penises that actually were so long or so large in diameter that they were uncomfortable. Some women made comments that men with average to shorted penises actually tried harder to please them and they appreciated that. The men with a stubby weren't conceited about their penis like many men with large ones. Penis conceit was not admired in the comments of most women. The Stubby doesn't work for the A-spot and if really short, won't work for the cervix. The stubby is especially good for bumping pubic bones and direct clitoral bumping which many women really seem to like. Men with a stubby are more effective sexual partners if they don't have a layer of fat on their pubic area which prevents firm bumping of pubic bones.

TORPEDO

This is a penis that has a smaller diameter at the base than at middle and at the end. This is a good shape for all stimulation except the A-spot (unless it is particularly long and then that works well also). It is sort of a combination of the mushroom and the stubby. It doesn't have as big of head as the mushroom, and the outer half is a stubby with the base more like a lance. This is a good all-purpose shape with no serious drawbacks, but no outstanding advantages.

TAPER

The taper is actually tapered in diameter from larger at the base and smaller at the head and with a rather small head with a minimal frenulum ridge around the head. This sounds like it would be unappealing, but it is a very effective shape for precise aiming. Since the head is small, the nerve endings are more concentrated and the heightened sensation can ping-pong back and forth between partners and add fuel to the fire. This is a good shape to stimulate the U-spot slowly and at just the right angle, is good for the G-spot if the penetration angle is right, good for targeting the cervix and if long enough is also good for the A-spot.

THE MONSTER

These are the really big ones—both long and large. Guys really are impressed with them as well as some women. My guess is that the women who especially like them have larger vaginas that require the large size for stimulation. Some women point out that most men with monsters are so impressed with themselves that think they are a gift to the world and they sometimes don't put much effort into technique to satisfy the woman. Women don't like that attitude. If you have a monster, be considerate of your mate, go slow and learn correct techniques so you won't be thought of as self-centered.

CIRCUMCISED OR NOT?

Just a quick mention of circumcised as opposed to uncircumcised men. Of course, any archetype of penis can be circumcised or not. It would seem that there might be a considerable difference between them due to the absence or presence of a foreskin. In the scant information I have found on the subject where women give their opinions, the difference is more a curiosity to women than a preference for one over the other. The presence or absence of a foreskin doesn't seem to make much difference to women's satisfaction. I include this statement just for the satisfaction of anyone's curiosity.

Now that we have gotten through the really graphic stuff, let's return to the more helpful relationship material.

INTERCOURSE

After you have had sex for several years (particularly with the same person), you are probably in a rut and you are both know and expect the same old things to happen. The adventure is gone. Sex has become a boring and predictable game of paint by numbers. You have experimented and practiced the same techniques on each other and it gets the job done, but you are likely bored to death. The excitement and the anticipation of adventure just isn't there anymore. Neither of you will say anything to the other for fear of a negative reaction and for fear of hurting the other person's feelings. That is something you have to change. Have a short frank discussion BEFORE and AFTER each sex session using the information I have described and openly discuss daring and quirky new positions, discuss things that even seem a little disgusting at first and be open minded. Don't beat it to death with long discussions that are uncomfortable, but discuss details enough to be titillating and to slowly make emotional headway. BE ADVENTUROUS AND DARING, but don't introduce too much at one time. Build on previous discussions and physical technique successes.

Use what you already know as the starting point. You will already know at least a couple of techniques that you have used successfully for years and they work on your partner. Use that as a starting point and slowly incorporate the things you weren't previously aware of or haven't ever tried before. If those have become stale and the old techniques don't work anymore, don't worry. That just tells you it is time for something new and adventurous. Just be very patient and be aware that habits are deeply ingrained and trying new things usually doesn't produce instant results. You will quickly become a true believer when a single new technique results in a new gleam in your partner's eye.

OPENLY DISCUSS SECRET SEXUAL DESIRES OR FANTASYS

This is an important sexual technique. Be candid with each other about those really secret things you always wanted to try. This is amazingly difficult and very uncomfortable at first. You will be surprised at the wild things your mate has already thought about, but has never dared to discuss. Being open and receptive with no recriminations. If something your partner says shocks you, contain your surprise and act as if it is completely ordinary to you. It sets a mood for fun and openness. Tell each other about some of your fantasies. Go slow at first and don't blurt out right away that you always wanted to have sex with a midget, a stranger with a huge penis, and two of your neighbors with a goat watching on your front lawn all at the same time. That much information all at once might shut the process down. Be prepared that some fantasies are a riot! The sexual fantasy of one man I had worked with long ago was to run barefoot through a roomful of "boobies". The dialogue should be edgy but not too shocking to start out. As the initial surprises become mutually evened out, you can slowly be even more open.

LEARN THE BASICS WITH ENTHUSIASM—HERE THEY ARE

In studying sex videos of numerous techniques, it is obvious that a few people are really into sex and they are the ones who get the most satisfactory results. Most others just lay there passively and use no hip motion, no leg movements and no muscular motion either in the penis or in the vagina and are unaware of the need for positioning their pubic bones in the exact relative position that allows the direct stimulation of all internal erogenous zones of the woman by using the woman's pubic bone as a fulcrum. Either the skilled man, or the skilled woman can guide the penis head to the exact spot, but they have to know about the way the penis is attached to the man and how it needs to be "sighted" to deliver the thrust to the precise spot. If both partners are highly knowledgeable and skilled, it becomes much easier.

In the missionary position, as the man's pubic bone is positioned upward in relation to the woman's pubic bone, the penis is directed more to the back of the vagina but closer to the urethra, the clitoral shield, and the U-spot. As the man's pubic bone is positioned lower in relation to the woman, the thrust is directed more upward to the anterior or front of the vagina where the erogenous sensations originate in all four G-spot zones, the cervix and the A-spot. The A-spot is easier to reach for a man with a slightly longer penis and if the woman positions her hips correctly with her legs bent and knees drawn up to her breasts, while she pumps her knees rhythmically with the penetration. As she curls her hips up and forward, the vagina will become taunt with deep thrusts and tug on the entire clitoral complex for a very fast and intense orgasm as the penis exerts pressure at the deepest part of the vagina and stimulates the A-spot on the way. The A-spot can also be reached by direct thrusts with the penis at a right angle to the vaginal vestibule (man standing position). All of this requires conscious activity and coordination that may be distracting at first, but soon becomes automatic. Men with a larger penis should be aware that they need to be careful not to put too much pressure against the deepest part of the woman's vagina. It can be painful if the man is careless. As the intensity builds, deeper thrusts directed at the A-spot are more acceptable to the woman and what at first was uncomfortable will become not only comfortable, but needed and requested. DO NOT RUSH IT! When she is ready for the really deep thrusts, you will know it. The man standing position thrusts the penis more directly against all of the interior erogenous zones as penetration occurs to different depths. The woman then is able to use her hip motion for fine and deadly accurate sighting of the penis to exactly where she wants it. She will have the fun and responsibility of precise control by using her hip scooping movements, the exact position of her pubic bone, and precise timing. This sounds as complicated as the verbal instructions for folding a box, but in practice, it is pretty easy after you both learn your vaginal geography.

If the woman curls her pelvis forward and up, and raises her hips off the bed with knees wide or rolls back and straightens her legs high in the air, she allows also a very deep penetration and full vaginal access which is good for the A-spot orgasm. Raising her feet upward as opposed to pointing her toes also enhances her sensations. The friction misses the clitoral head directly, but allows for a more accessible inner vaginal stimulation. It also stimulates the erectile bulbs of the clitoral root which indirectly stimulates the entire clitoral complex as the deep penetration tugs at the full length of the vagina. The action can be altered to change between every erogenous spot by either or both partners momentarily scooting up or down against each other by small amounts so that the penis is aimed exactly at what really feels good at the moment. The sensation for the man is also enhanced by the woman using her heels to grab behind his thighs and pull him forcefully into her pubic bone. (Also, ladies, speaking of heels, most men asked are really turned on by high heels in bed even if you are wearing nothing else). The female's thigh contractions and the additional pressure pulling you together enhance the pleasure for both partners. The tension of the leg muscles isolates the erogenous impulses inside the woman and the obvious active participation is a VERY potent cheering signal for the man. I have yet to see or participate in any sex session that is only mediocre when the woman actively uses her hips, legs and overall body movement to enhance both her and her partner's stimulation.

THE FORMULA FOR A POOR SEX LIFE

The sure way to have a poor to mediocre sex life is to just lay there staring at the ceiling while your mind is somewhere else. The man can be no better than the woman sets the stage for. If you want a failed sex life, women, just spread your legs and lay there motionless with the attitude that you want it to end as soon as possible. Men if you want to destroy your sex life and your marriage, be rough, selfish and demanding of your mate.

WHAT MEN WANT---WHAT WOMEN WANT

Men like WIGGLE and men like ENTHUSIASM. Some very homely women instantly become very sexy simply with their enthusiasm, confidence and skillful hip movements. Most men would take a skilled and enthusiastic lover over a beauty queen. My guess is that women would also choose a skilled lover over a hunk any day. The beauty is lost on the eyes. We all enjoy looking at a beautiful member of the opposite sex, but many of those beauties are so full of themselves that they think they only have to show up rather than to know much or work at doing much. They might just think they are so special that they are doing you a favor to allow you to experience them while their actual skills may be lacking. Some people that I have known are so accustomed to such automatic positive responses, that they don't even attempt to hone their personalities or even their manners. I hope your mate is not one of those. That is not to just categorize them, because I know many extraordinarily physically beautiful people who are also fine people in every other way and their beauty didn't spoil them. I am just saying that beauty and sexual skills are not related. Anyone can become a highly desirable and skilled sexual being and that can overcome the absence of physical beauty alone.

Women have expressed the desire in many diversified studies for MEN TO SLOW DOWN AND TO PAY ATTENTION TO THE PHYSICAL AND PSYCHOLOGICAL NEEDS OF THEIR MATE. One of the overall universal complaints is that men seem to be focused on their own pleasure and immediate needs and the woman is just the means to fulfill those needs. Women want to feel included as a part of a loving and respectful relationship. If men would get it through their heads that the magic speed of .8 Hertz (slightly slower than one movement per second) is one of the keys to stimulate their mates the most efficiently, some of that complaint would be solved. That goes from penetrating strokes of a penis, dildo, or fingers to tongue movements to sucking movements on the woman's nipples. I STRESS THAT

IT IS AN UNNATURALLY SLOW PACE AND HAS TO BE CONSCIOUSLY LEARNED. That is why I have explained it and mentioned it over and over in so many places throughout the book.

THE POSITION OF CONTROL FOR A WOMAN

In the cowgirl positions (both forward and reverse), the woman has most of the control to use her front to back hip movements. The movements can be either smooth and rhythmic or jerkier, to completely control the penis thrust or even positioning herself downward on the man so that his penis bends around the pubic bone and directly rubs the clitoral head and sheath. In several studies, the cowgirl positions are preferred by many women. The societal roll of women has changed and I think that women are more sexually aggressive today and the cowgirl positions allows for their liberation to be more manifest. It's about time! Hooray for women's equality! Many men really are turned on by the view of beautiful breasts swaying and bouncing at a convenient viewing angle as the woman gently undulates at center stage over them.

HIP SCOOPING AGAIN-----REALLY?---- ENOUGH ALREADY!

In the cowgirl positions, the motion of the woman should NOT be raising herself up and down with the legs. That is one of the first signs of a poorly skilled woman. Instead it should be a sliding forward and backward motion using hip thrusting and scooping. Let's forever call this "hip scooping". I have mentioned it here and several other places in the book because it is so important. It is highly effective for both partners when done well. It is a restful position that can be with the woman vertical in cowgirl position or horizontally laying on top of the man and for her to be in complete control without getting crushed. Cowgirl position has the added benefit of gravity working as an enhancement because the internal female parts tend to drop down a bit toward the action particularly if she is in the vertical position of the cowgirl.

A REALLY FUN ALTERNATE POSITION

The "doggie" position I have referred to previously is the favorite of some men because of the erotic view of the woman and her heart shaped rear end. He can also watch the penetration and watch as the woman produces lubricative juices which can be highly erotic. Doggie position is used for both vaginal intercourse, and also by the more adventurous for anal intercourse. I will caution here once again. Once anal penetration occurs, re-entry into the vagina without thorough bacterial cleansing can cause a vaginal infection. Don't do that! Additionally, anal intercourse is illegal in some states and is considered unacceptable or immoral by many. I'm not sure how homosexuality can be condoned and legal, but anal intercourse condemned at the same time. The next decades will answer that. In any case, cleanliness is paramount.

Doggie position allows again for the knowledgeable woman to use her hip motion to direct the penis exactly where she wants it control the stimulation any way she wants it, but she has to be aware that she has that control and responsibility when she takes that position. It is her expertise that determines the outcome. Her hip angle is her control and changing her hip angle is key to both partner's stimulation by arching her back downward and then humping up her back. Physical therapists call this motion camel/cat exercises. One interesting and highly erotic sensation can be achieved by the woman who is on her hands and knees to drop her stomach and arch her back downward like a swayback horse to allow air entry into the vagina and the man to penetrate which gives a very stimulating "touch and touch break" sensation as the man's penis head barely contacts and breaks contact with various spots in the inflated and open vagina as he flexes his penis. It is surprisingly unique and stimulating sensation.

HULA DANCERS, BELLY DANCERS, AND STRIPPERS

I have concentrated so far on the woman's use of her hips tilted forward and backward to hit the perfect spots. Now let's get more sophisticated and add even more to the scooping motion. The technique that has been used to describe professional strippers for decades----the "bump and grind" is very effective and erotic. This is distinctly different than the tilting and rocking motions of hip scooping. The grind is a rotational motion of the hips similar to the motion to a hula dancer or the slower rhythm of the famous "Hula Hoop" toy many of us used as kids. In addition to being visually sensual, it is also an important motion to learn for G-spot stimulation during intercourse and for cervical stimulation. This is the wiggle. The "bump" is the jerky off axis motion of the hips at random which introduces unpredictability into the motion mix. Think of some of the Latin dances. These motions are all usable by both partners at unpredictable times to enhance the sex. Sometimes the predictability of a rhythmic motion unexpectedly interrupted by a wiggle or a thrust out of rhythm can cause instant orgasm. It adds more fun and unpredictability into the mix. I once saw a really skilled world class stripper in a beachfront night club in Rio de Janeiro that was the epitome of the bump and grind motion and, wow, what a skill. That was 40 years ago and it is still fresh in my mind. She was feminine elegance at its best and it was all visual. I have seen some very overweight women who were packing some wrinkles and saggy parts who were just as enticing as they gyrated. Women, it is up to you. Any woman who learns that skill or some belly dancing skills and uses them in the bedroom does herself and her mate a real service. It is all designed to be a turn on and it is. It all sets the mood for a magic carpet adventure.

AN ANGEL IN PUBLIC AND A DEMON IN BED

There is an old saying that "men want their wives to be an angel in public and a demon in bed!" Don't take this literally, but you get the point. BE RESPONSIVE physically and verbally AND BE UNINHIBITED. I will say that again--- BE RESPONSIVE AND BE UNINHIBITED. Allow your passion to show and become noisy in bed. Continually be aware of "allowing" sex to be fun rather than trying to "make" it fun. The more uninhibited you become, the more fun and satisfaction you will have. Take every opportunity to show enthusiastic interest and appreciation for all of your mate's body parts and express it to them in detailed words.

HAND JOBS

Unless you are a real neophyte ladies, you know what a hand job is. The thing is that you probably never learned how to do it right. Your mate was probably just glad that you would even do it, so he finally orgasmed with the most rudimentary of stimulation. The usual depiction of a hand job is with the woman using her lubricated hands to make a tube with her fingers wrapped around her partner's penis and pump up and down. A good hand job entails sexy and suggestive talking. Complete rolling massage of the entire genital area including the scrotum, hand over hand tugging and wrapping, cupping the palms into a pocket and rolling them all around his frenulum and penis head, tickling around the ridge at the head of the penis, lightly stretching the head in a rhythmic motion, very gently rubbing the testicles and an expert sense of timing to know when to stop the stimulation just before orgasm and let him settle down a little in repeated cycles so that the experience goes on and on for him and he doesn't orgasm. Keep him at this state just under orgasm until he tells you to kick him over. These techniques are also very effective used in combination with a blow job.

The secret is the "tease". The rise and fall of the level of stimulation is where the real pleasure is for him. Men being very visual creatures are having their mind run wild with anticipation as you skillfully tease him into orgasm, slowly and tantalizingly.

Hand jobs are easy and very powerful when a "quickie" is just the thing. You'd be surprised how effective they are when you offer them unexpectedly.

MISSIONARY AIN'T BORING

Any time the "missionary" face to face position is discussed, it always seems to be with a hint of boredom. I don't feel that way. It is the position that is the most conducive to kissing, verbal communication and the best position to look your mate directly in the eyes and into their soul. It is also highly effective if you know about hip motion and relative pubic bone placement. It can allow for the most body contact between partners which can be one of the most satisfying parts of sex.

I personally think that there is too much emphasis on possible positions for intercourse and maybe that is because I haven't tried each possible one, but my wife and I have tried enough different positions to realize that for us at least, the secret of success is more about technique than dozens of positions of the Kama Sutra.

SEX FOR VARIETY AND SEX FOR POST ERECTILE COUPLES

Since intercourse has already been addressed, and it is truly wonderful, but there are a large majority of older couples that deal with the reality that erections for them are in the past. It can be caused from any number of problems ranging from various medical conditions to the medicines used to treat them. Up until now, many of those people just gave up and let their sex lives wither away, along with the spark in their personalities. That is no longer appropriate because a very adventurous and active sex life exists for ANYONE if they will put out a diligent and consistent effort. NEWS FLASH FOR THOSE THAT MISSED IT PREVIOUSLY-----MEN and WOMEN don't need erections in the mix for the men or for the women to achieve advanced level orgasms including multiple orgasms and female ejaculation for the woman! MEN CAN ORGASM WITHOUT AN ERECTION, and the orgasm is just as strong as orgasm with an erection.

ERECTILE DYSFUNCTION CAN BE A HIDDEN BLESSING

In some ways erectile dysfunction is a major blessing because a man can perform more precise and enduring stimulation to his mate with a dildo for longer periods than he ever could with his penis. He may have a compromised heart and simply not have the stamina to thrust for long periods. He can also give his partner the experiential answer to the question "Does size matter?" if he isn't a tightwad and is willing to buy a few different sizes and shapes of dildos for her. (Yes, men ---- despite what they will initially admit to, all women-- including your wife-- has pondered that question, but I doubt that she would have admitted it). Women who are blessed with a large clitoris with an erectile shaft and men who are blessed with a larger penis do have some advantage but not so large an advantage that skill isn't much more important. It just makes some positions and techniques somewhat easier for them.

The other benefit which is really important using a dildo is that a man can position himself sitting between his partners' legs and closely observe delicate twitches, hip motions, smells, and secretions which are the observable responses to his stimulation using the dildo and finger or thumb stimulation on her clitoral head, or instead use a separate clitoral vibrator simultaneously with the dildo. He can direct the dildo internally exactly to the target erotic spot and easily control the timing, touch, intensity and depth of the thrust or gentle motion with precision. He can learn to read all of her subtle micro-movements and guide her sexual response with finesse. This is a combination training exercise for the man and an awakening exercise for the woman to awaken dormant feedback circuits.

AWAKENING DORMANT SEXUAL CIRCUITS

Once again, it is pleasurable erotic experimentation that awakens dormant or atrophied circuits, adds foreplay and anticipation to the mix, and adds spice to a stale and previously predictable encounter. As a man learns his mate's vaginal geography he will become more astute and exponentially more effective. He will become skilled by systematically directing specific attention to awakening sensations that have been buried and dormant in his mate for many years, or erotic triggers that never have been awakened because the woman's experience had never included them in her first sexual experiences. If she had trained herself to rely on direct clitoral stimulation alone for satisfaction then she simply didn't know that there was anything else to experience. This experimentation using a dildo and a separate clitoral vibrator is actually the very best way for the man to educate himself and then to relay what he is experiencing to his partner. She can then correlate what he is describing to what her sensations are. That mental picture he verbally provides for her becomes her new standard and becomes the starting gun for her arousal. Her responses will be a mix of voluntary and involuntarily. Each session becomes a bio-feedback experience where she learns to actually control her responses and make the necessary mental and physical associations which will bring her long dormant circuits to life. After diligent practice, the man can become so good at actually reading the woman's sensations by her micro movements transmitted THROUGH the dildo, that he is able to move her sensations from one area to another at will, thereby orchestrating different kinds of orgasms for her at will. When a woman is aroused, she creates many different micro-movements that tell her mate exactly what is happening inside her, but he has to know how to interpret those signals through the dildo. That will be addressed in a few paragraphs below.

LEARN THE MELODY OF HER TRIGGERS

The woman becomes more precious to a man because she is a skilled and trained partner and he becomes more precious to her for the very same reason. This becomes one of the most erotic experiences possible when the man realizes exactly which tiny motions trigger her response and he is able to literally "play" her vagina like a musician plays their musical instrument. Some erectile dysfunctional men have been known to respond to this exercise with an unexpected erection because the exercise itself is highly erotic to both partners. Female hormones are released from the vaginal area and since the man's nose is closer to the source, he will be more aware of them. The sensing of her hormones alone sometimes is the only trigger necessary to cause an erection. When a woman realizes that she has the control over her vaginal response, she is further aroused and the process creates a feedback loop until at least one orgasm occurs and she will usually not want to stop right then. Don't be surprised that after the man learns to read tiny responses through a dildo, the woman won't want to stop after having just one orgasm, but wants to continue further stimulation or additional orgasms or to hold at a very heightened near orgasmic state after the initial orgasm. Successive orgasms can target other vaginal triggers for even deeper fulfillment. Some of the most fun experiences occur after the first orgasm is out of the way and she is still in a highly aroused state. It is the launching platform for the second stage booster. Some women report that their orgasms even increase in intensity after having a clitoral or combination orgasm and then subsequent G-spot or A-spot orgasms. Again, each of these orgasms are distinctly different. Combination orgasms seem to help in opening the circuits to all other specific zones. Each zone seems to relax and become receptive to the proper stimulation and the high level of arousal can continue until either one of the partners decided to close the curtain and stop. At that stage the woman can go into an altered state where she seems to be floating in the sensations with eyes rolled back. All vaginal muscles relax and everything is in perfect synchronicity. She will let you know when she can't take any more and is too exhausted to continue. She can go into a state where all else is completely blocked out and she remains lost in her highly aroused state as long as you continue the slow and gentle stimulation.

GUYS, YOU ARE IN THE DRIVER'S SEAT-- PAY ATTENTION— WATCH THESE SPECIFIC MICRO-MOVEMENTS

All of this is depends on the man being able to read her very subtle responses and micro-movements. He must continue the stimulation with exactly the right response after she has learned to awaken her sexual circuits to each erogenous zone. This takes time and dedication, but once you experience it, you'll think all of the effort was worth it. When you get to this point in your skill level, your sexual bond will be stronger than ever. Pay particular attention to color changes in different vaginal zones as blood flow increases, tiny changes in the texture or color of the nipples and areolas, erection and wrinkling of the nipples and areolas, note the throbbing in her neck as her heartbeat increases, and become an expert at interpreting the twitching of all of the muscles surrounding her vagina, in her legs, in her stomach muscles, and the movement of her toes. Watch for the starting and for changes in her vaginal secretions. Some are slick and clear, some are milky, some are ropey with a syrupy consistency and some have particulates in them. Feel the G-spot and note the textural and erectile changes. Listen carefully and learn to interpret all of her personal sounds. She will have moaning and cooing sounds. Carefully watch her micro facial expressions. Some of them are very subtle but tell you a lot. Watch for subtle muscular movements around the eyes and mouth. Feel for PC muscle flexing and vertical vaginal muscle twitches just inside the vagina. BE OBSERVANT! Micro-movements are just that---- micro---- small and barely perceptible especially until you get used to them.

If you are a man with a fully functioning rock hard penis and that is the only tool you have, I kind of feel sorry for you. You might think you have it all, but you don't. Your male ego will be inseparably tied to your penis and you might be reluctant to opening your mind to the things you think you know, but don't. You are missing some of the best learning experiences about vaginal geography that can only be learned by stimulating your mate with a dildo or with your fingers. If a hard penis is all you know, you are also depriving your mate of several different and potent and extended forms of orgasmic bliss. Put out the effort to expand your horizons. A hard penis is great, but it is far from everything.

(See the section on the use of dildos by the man on his partner which I will expand on more a few pages later.)

ORAL SEX MIGHT BE OLDER AND MORE COMPLEX THAN YOU THINK

We post-menopausal folks grew up in a world where many of us were taught that oral sex was very much a fringe subject and most of us were passively taught that it was somehow "edgy" at best and disgusting at worst. Oral sex has been routinely and enthusiastically practiced in cultures all over the world for thousands of years. It only was burdened with a negative connotation through hypocritical officials who wanted to secretly practice it, but condemn it for the common populous.

Oral sex is one of the most satisfying and intimate forms of sex and it can be practiced by anyone. Even by couples dealing with erectile dysfunction. It is treated openly and positively in all books I have seen devoted to human sexuality. Basic instinct pretty well gets you started, but unfortunately, that instinctual level only takes you to about the sixth grade level of expertise in sex training school. To go further, we need some advanced tips for both fellatio and cunnilingus.

THE TONGUE IS A MARVELOUS AND DEXTROUS INSTRUMENT

The tongue is an extremely versatile and precise instrument with exactly the right muscular control and the precisely the right combination of textures. The top of the tongue is covered by individual bumps called taste buds and is perfect for creating the precisely controlled friction on the eyeball sensitive female clitoral head and the ultra-sensitive male frenulum and ridge around the penile head. The smooth underside of the tongue is perfect for the opposite sensations of a smooth gentle motion with little friction, and the little skin attachment under the tongue (also called frenulum) both provide additional vital variations to the wonderful tongue as a sex tool. The tongue has a full range of motions that allows unlimited stimulating ability. It is an absolutely perfect instrument of sexual pleasure for both genders if you train yourself to use it well.

The tongue can be used in a darting motion, a flattened side to side motion (using the top or bottom surface), a flicking motion, a circular motion, and for pressure motions. Unlike an erect penis, it is highly controllable and able to change to many shapes with infinite combinations of motion. Unlike a vagina, it can deliver precise stimulation exactly where and how you want it delivered to your mate, and unlike a penis, it is extremely deft. It is an absolutely indispensable tool for the sexual tool box.

FELLATIO

Any woman who is wanting to become a highly prized sexual partner will increase her sexual worth several fold by pointedly learning how to perform fellatio or blowjobs well. Just as in intercourse, it isn't difficult to stumble through the act and arrive at a climax, but that once again, is a very low bar to set for yourself. Most women simply put part or all of the penis in their mouth and pump in and out. That is boring to men and even though it produces an orgasm, it isn't one that is likely to be remembered. That level of skill is the precursor to the man developing a wandering eye. Your goal is to plant memories of fantastic sessions with YOU as an ENTHUSIASTIC, EXPERIMENTAL, AND FULLY ATTENTIVE SEXUAL PARTNER that will be remembered for years. You distinguish yourself to that degree by becoming the most skilled at making him feel like he is revered. His fragile male ego requires it and his constantly replenishing hormones require it. Those memories create lasting bonds that cement relationships on a deep mental, physical and emotional level. Many women don't view themselves as sexual prizes, but that is completely up to your willingness to devote your efforts to your mate in a way that it is impossible for him to think of you as anything but a prize that he treasures. Use both the coarsely textured top side of your tongue, the tip of your tongue and the smooth bottom side of your tongue to stimulate the whole penis head and particularly the cleft or frenulum on the bottom side of the head. Also use the different parts of your tongue to stimulate the sensitive ridge around the head of the penis. Experiment with various pressures, speeds and combinations. Don't forget to gently massage the scrotum and illicit verbal responses from him as to what is feeling the best to him.

BE INNOVATIVE, EXPERIMENTAL AND UNPREDICTABLE

The pizazz in all sexual fun is the anticipation, the staging, the teasing, and then the skillful increase in unpredictable stimulation. The slam, bam, thank you ma'am won't be memorable. On the other hand, a carefully timed orchestrated series of textural changes, pressures, vacuum action, and mouth pressures of various kinds, accompanied by gentle scrotal massage and caresses will create a lasting memory in your mate's mind that will keep him at home wanting more and wanting to fully satisfy you in any way you want, both inside and outside the bedroom. BE INNOVATIVE and be experimental and unpredictable. That will cure any boredom. Try VERY gently tugging on his testicles and use your hands to isolate the feeling on the penis. Try stretching the skin snugly over the end as you use combinations of tongue techniques. In short, try anything that comes to mind. Make his penis feel like it is the master of ceremonies at the Super Bowl. Picture in your mind what it might feel like to him as you perform your symphony and view yourself as experiencing your stimulation as is it was happening to you instead of to him. Imagine the same motions on your clitoris and it will turn you on at the same time. Mentally switching places with him and try to experience the event through your partner is extremely helpful in building excitement. Also mentally think about how the feeling you are producing in him corresponds to what various vaginal penetrations for him would feel like. That is what he is doing. Be in the moment and be engrossed in now. Slip in and out of a few fantasies of your own and use your biggest sex instrument---your brain to imagine anything that is erotic to you as you are stimulating him. BE ENTHUSIASTIC! If you want a really tame and loving husband, this is the way to do it.

If you are new to oral sex, an obvious question is how to handle the ejaculate. It is loaded with human testosterone which is a very expensive and precious natural hormone. Women have some testosterone as well as men and it is the hormone that induces sexual desire for women and men alike. Some women smear it on their skin for quick absorption and a later sexual desire boost when it is absorbed. Some women swallow it, and some women try to avoid it because it is messy. Do whatever makes sense to you. Most women find that the involuntary contractions of the man during ejaculation is a turn on and they want to retain at least some of the ejaculate. Testosterone laden male ejaculate is an effective anti-wrinkle cream.

The tongue is a wonderful instrument. Learn to use it with skill and always be guided by your partners' responses. Learn to read very, very subtle sounds, hip actions, thrusts, twitches. You will soon find that each of his responses will enhance your own pleasure you will literally become one with him. The two of you will feel united and bonded closer than ever before. What could be better for a lasting marriage and physical, financial, mental and emotional security?

P.S. Don't forget to use your lips in your experimentation. Watch a horse eat a carrot or an apple.

CUNNILINGUS

Some women are concerned about how they smell down there, but any healthy person who bathes daily will only have healthy smells. If either partner has any hang-ups, just go wash and rinse the area well. Some people like perfume, but many like me and Napoleon, prefer a la natural. Notwithstanding, the back side must be sparklingly clean.

Being between your mate's thighs with your tongue exploring her every bump and hollow of her vaginal area puts all of your senses right at mission control with a center stage view. At 70 plus, I'm still discovering new territory. You can see minute details of texture, and shapes that you have looked at hundreds of times, but swear you never noticed before. (I think women metamorphose daily so they can surprise us!) In this position you can smell the distinctly feminine scents of all four of the different vaginal secretions as they are released during stimulation. You can feel and see mini-twitching involuntary reactions to your stimulating efforts and you can be engulfed in the super musky aromas of female hormones and pheromones. It is quite an encompassing experience once you are knowledgeable enough to marvel at what is really happening literally under your nose. This and the next section about the use of dildos is a very important training regimen that will really open you up to how much you have to learn even after spending many years thinking you already know most there is to know.

Men, think of your tongue and lips as the highly controllable and sensitive instruments that they are. Creatively think to yourself "How many different ways can I imagine to use these instruments to bring pleasure to every part of my mate? What would possibly feel good to her"? Then dig in, start experimenting, and let your mind picture what is happening inside her body as you start to see and feel her micro-movements. If you are doing anything right, you will start to see, feel, and smell her body kick in as she responds to your touches. Be sensitive to her tiny movements which signal what is really turning her on. Learn to read her every movement, no matter how small. Sometimes those responsive movements are hard to read and you have to be mentally present, absorbed, and in the game. It is all about setting up a feedback loop of her neural signals to her brain and creating an "echo" of stimulation which builds very slightly upon the previous neural signal. Those tiny twitches in the vertical pencil sized muscles on the outer sides of the vagina, tiny leg twitches, and clitoral head engorgement and erection are all screaming to you that you need to continue what you are doing. THINK ONLY ABOUT HER SATISFACTION and not your own. My guess is that you are already getting plenty of satisfaction in doing what you are doing. Use your own mind to imagine exactly what she is feeling and remember EXACTLY what turns her on for next time and mix that into other new and different maneuvers. Listen very carefully to any sounds she makes. Some women are loud and some are extremely subtle. Are you getting the picture----sex is mental as well as physical. All women are different and each has personal preferences. Try any and all techniques during several different sessions. What works one time might need to be altered the next time you try it. Learn to use the texture differences of the top and bottom of your tongue and learn to point the end for darting into any tiny recesses she finds pleasurable. You will be surprised at your versatility. Clitoral head stimulation is a biggie, the area around the clitoral sheath is a biggie, the opening of the urethra is a biggie and the U-spot area around the urethral opening is a biggie. All of them require a different touch.

THE MAGICAL FREQUENCY OF ORGASMIC CONTRACTIONS

Remember for about the tenth time, that orgasmic contractions are at .8 Hertz or slightly slower than one per second, and to get to orgasm, it is very useful to maintain that rate for tongue movement. Side to side movement over the general clitoral area and just underneath it with the top of a flattened tongue with significant pressure is very effective when done at .8 hertz. It will seem extremely slow as you are doing it, but mentally time your movements and keep them slowed down. It is extremely effective when done right. The natural tendency is to allow the speed of stimulating movements to keep speeding up and you will find that you have to make a very conscious effort to keep tongue movements slowed to barely slower than one per second. When she starts verbally "cooing", you will know it is time to settle in on what you are doing and stop searching. You'll know what I mean when you hear the sounds. Most women do it involuntarily and don't even know they are doing it. Sometimes you can kick in the afterburner by slightly, and I mean only slightly, altering your tongue movements temporarily from the .8 hertz to either .9 hertz, or .7 hertz just for a stroke or two. The slight change of very slightly slowing or speeding the stimulation will often bring on orgasm within a couple of seconds if done just at the right time. Also a very brief pausing for a second or two also jolts her when she reaches a plateau near orgasm but is stuck at that level and can't quite orgasm. Always respond to any verbal comments from her by holding a steady course as long as she responds. Do EXACTLY what she wants. When you get really practiced at reading her micro-movements, her secretions, and watch the stimulating rate, you will be able to bounce along just below orgasm for long periods and she will be in ecstasy until YOU decide to kick her into orgasm. After a session of this, she will be what I will call very agreeable for at least half a day. After two of these, she won't get out of bed for a day, and she won't even care that you didn't take out the trash.

One additional tip---use cunnilingus along with the finger techniques described in the next paragraph together for a double whammy. It is a little awkward physically for the man to do all at once, but it is a really good ride for her! You'll think you are a champion rodeo rider if you can ride her all the way through orgasm while she is shoving down on your head because the sensation is so intense for her. If she can ride it out, a second orgasm is usually inevitable.

SQUIRTING (FEMALE EJACULATION) IS A VITAL SKILL

This is an extremely important skill and phenomenon that most people over 50 didn't know about and still don't. It is misunderstood by many gynecologists and was only really widely witnessed in sex videos after the internet was in wide use. Some of the encounters are faked, but most are very real. As time goes on and more people become aware of the real thing, a higher percentage appear to be real rather than faked as more people see the real thing and learn about it.

It is a vital skill that men need to learn to be able to wake up their partner's G-spot circuits, and women need to know for themselves. It usually involves the vigorous stimulation of the general G-spot area by the man using either one or two fingers usually rapidly rubbing in and out of the vagina with forward firm pressure against the lower inside edge and back side of the pubic bone. The stimulating fingers (one or two) are curved around and behind the pubic bone. There are some instructional videos available for the technique and the men who know how to do it well are highly desirable sex partners because of it. I personally prefer a more specific approach after learning about the 4 different G-spot zones and concentrating on individual zones, but both approaches work. The most important thing about it is that UNTIL A WOMAN HAS A TRULY GENUINE SQUIRTING EXPERIENCE OF REAL SKENES FLUID, SHE HASN'T FOUND AND AWAKENED HER G-SPOT. It took my wife and me nearly 6 years of trying in many, many short sessions to make it work. The final result was that she was able to achieve the very strong G-spot orgasm accompanied by female ejaculation. After the initial success, she trained her body to respond through repeated stimulations creating a positive mental circuit biofeedback loop to an area that was dormant her whole life because she didn't know anything about it. Her G-spot slowly started to awaken fully, zone by zone until all four areas were highly functional. When a particular pleasure is remembered each time, the memory reinforces the expectation of another pleasurable experience and at some point, the response becomes activated and the circuits are completed to make the response automatic. She is now highly orgasmic in all four G-spot sub areas. (I celebrated her achievement by giving her some 18 karat gold drop gold earrings from Tiffany's. We refer to these as her "squirting" earrings and she is very proud of them privately). This skill is critical. Female ejaculation is the door to awakening up other dormant internal vaginal circuits and in erasing the damage caused by long term inhibitions or negative imprinting. The stimulation is described by some adept men as being more of a very firm pressure or tapping on the inside of the pubic bone and it is truly exhausting for the man because the pressure is very firm and the rhythm is fast (a harmonic of the .8 Hertz), but if you hit just the right spot, her eyes will begin to roll. This single exception is where it is sometimes necessary to use a very rapid stimulation as opposed to the base .8 Hertz rate. It also helps to press down on her bladder area just above her pubic bone with your other hand as you are positioned at her side. It is pretty intense and you will find that you have to do it intermittently because you will fatigue quickly. As soon as her orgasm starts and she squirts, she will grab your hand to remove the pressure so she can finish her squirting ejaculation. Be sure to have a couple of towels under her because the volume of her ejaculate can be profuse.

The naysayers of female ejaculation, including some medical people, claim that the fluid squirted out is urine since it is expelled from the urethra. Anyone who is actually skilled in the technique will assure you that genuine female ejaculation is not urine, although a very tiny amount of urine can leak in and is sometimes present. The Skene's fluid empties into the urethra near the opening, so it comes out the same place as urine. The fluid varies from a light honey color with a syrupy consistency, to translucent milky, to more colorless and is astringent. It sometimes has some suspended cloudy specks and streaks in it. Sometimes it is just a few drops which ooze out and sometimes an ejaculating intermittent squirt occurs, and sometimes a high pressure squirt which shoots several feet. Different women have a different response pattern which can even vary from one orgasm to another. The volume varies from a few drops to a pint or so and I have heard of as much as a quart. Some multi orgasmic women actually dehydrate themselves doing it with multiple orgasms. When you practice it, you might want to put down a piece of plastic sheeting on the bed and have a couple of washcloths and towels to absorb the liquid.

There have been some studies on the fluid and it is considered by most researchers that it is similar to male prostatic fluid produced by the Skene's glands located under the surface of the G-spot and the vigorous stimulation of the G-spot causes what is known as the female ejaculation. True Skene's fluid has a mild and rather neutral smell and the genuine ejaculate does not smell at all like urine. Urine is usually slightly yellow and smells like urine. The skeins gland itself is the bump you are feeling when you stimulate the G-spot in the #3 position. During initial contact, arousal and orgasm, the entire G-spot area, including all four parts, continually changes by engorging, flattening, wrinkling and smoothing out sometimes over and over again depending on the rate of stimulation, the pressure and the specific motion. It is pretty fascinating to feel. Learning to read these changes is part of learning her own unique micro-movements.

Some women require very vigorous and rapid stimulation for female ejaculation. The process is quite intense with an extremely intense and dramatic orgasm resulting which is accompanied by a strongly strained expulsive vaginal muscular response and very emotional involuntary quaking and verbal exclamations including squealing or screaming. Many of these women urgently require multiple consecutive G-spot orgasms before they reach complete satisfaction and they are not at all bashful about telling you in a very urgent tone. Others have a more tamed response with intermittent small squirts and extremely strong internal PC muscle contractions at .8 hertz. All are followed by an extreme letdown phase. The women with a more tamed response appear to respond better to a less vigorous and rhythmic stimulation and a side to side or circular motion with the fingers rubbing across the bump of the Skene's glands under the G-spot #2 and #3 position, or to a come hither curling of the stimulating fingers on the #2 and #3 G-spot position (the #3 position is the area of the cross ridges of her G-spot in most women). Try varying pressures and varying rhythms. When a response initiates, it is strong, usually sudden and not at all subtle. The exact combination of stimulation has to be found for each woman. It is like picking a lock in the sense that it is a complete failure until the second it happens, but when the lock is picked correctly, it opens quickly. In other words, expect her to go from zero to 100 miles per hour and hit orgasm in just a very few seconds. The first success can be really stubborn, but each successive time becomes easier after the first success. G-spot orgasms which are accompanied by female ejaculation are usually very strong and can induce a catatonic like dazed response that is one of the best sensations a woman can experience. The only thing remotely comparable for a man is a prostate combination orgasm.

ANAL STIMULATION

Anal stimulation is training of the erogenous structure of the anus either using a finger or with a wide variety of sex toys which were invented with a unique shape for that purpose. If it is something that appeals to you after the initial shock of the idea, you will likely find that there is more to know than you had ever thought. There is a longitudinal ridge inside the anus which is highly sensitive. It is located about 1 to 2 inches inside past the anal sphincter on the front wall of the anal canal and positioned just behind the G-spot of the vagina in women. It is fugitive, which means that it appears and disappears and changes texture at different points in the stimulating and orgasmic phase. It is connected to everything else in a woman's pelvic area and responds to direct slow, and very gentle stimulation. Start with the orgasmic frequency of .8 Hertz or barely slower than one movement per second. It is sometimes the trigger that works when other stimulation isn't working and she is slow to respond. If stimulated correctly, the resulting orgasm rivals or exceeds a strong G-spot orgasm but is distinctly different with a more encompassing general pelvic letdown phase and with a possibly even deeper and more general feeling of total satisfaction. The stimulation should be extremely slow, rhythmic, and extremely gentle using the texture of your fingerprint for just the perfect amount of friction. Some people use a finger cot and the difference in sensation using one of them is similar to the difference in using a condom or not using one during intercourse. You lose the fingerprint stimulation with a finger cot.

Always practice good hygiene afterward and DO NOT TOUCH ANYTHING ELSE including any other part of your mate until you thoroughly sterilize your finger or any other toy you might use. Always remember that internal anal tissue is very delicate and should always be lubricated with a water based personal lubricant.

THE ELUSIVE SEARCH FOR THE "WHOLE BODY ORGASM"

As mentioned previously, there is such a thing as a whole body orgasm and it is a remarkably impressive thing to see. I have seen five of them experienced by five different women in recorded sexual encounters and they are extremely intense. The women are completely uninhibited, uncontrollable, and in an alternate consciousness during the actual orgasm. At the end of the orgasm, they are totally exhausted and limp in the letdown phase and are almost unable to move for a short time. During this time they react by wildly repelling any further stimulation of their erogenous zones and do not want to be touched in any way for several seconds. They appear to require the expenditure of at least two or three times the orgasmic energy that a really good, normal G-spot/clitoral combination orgasm and the corresponding exhaustion at letdown. Unfortunately, whole body orgasms are as rare as hens' teeth and it seems that only a very few women are able to experience them. They involve a completely uncontrollable quaking of the entire body with an extreme and urgent imperative need to stop all stimulation instantly after the orgasm has started. If you ever see one or have one, it is unmistakable. They seem to be the result of an extremely uninhibited and enthusiastic woman stimulated by a really expert level partner who is highly skilled in giving G-spot orgasms at will. Just know there is such a thing, so in the unlikely event that your mate has one, you didn't really kill her, she just has to have some time to recover without being touched. If she does ever have one, she deserves a four hour rest, a hand engraved trophy and the best dinner money can buy. If you ever see one, you will never forget it.

USING DILDOS BY THE MAN ON HIS PARTNER ***A KEY EXERCISE***

This practice is some of the most important practice you can do. If you are persistent, you and your partner will learn more about sex from this exercise than any other form. As wonderful as the penis is, it can't begin to compete with a skillfully used dildo for stamina, accuracy, or the ability of the user to observe tiny responses that are viewed close up in real time. The typical positions of intercourse simply don't allow the same observation and deftness.

There are any number of dildos available for order through the internet or in sex toy shops in any city. They range from actual castings of real penises to enormous sized versions or fantasy versions which are more humorous than practical. The best ones are actual real life castings in cyberskin which is a type of properly flesh colored soft but firm silicone rubber/PVC material which is a very lifelike in both texture and flexibility. If you close your eyes and touch cyberskin, you will think you are touching real flesh. It is totally realistic, very durable and with care will last many years. I have done considerable experimentation with many of these and have settled on three different ones which seem to work the best when that is the kind of stimulation we want to use in that session.

YOU MAY WANT TO CUSTOMIZE

The first thing I discovered is that the vibrator that is imbedded in many of the cyberskin dildos is totally useless and each one had to be modified by removing the vibrator capsule and using the remaining cavity in the center to superglue a 3/8 inch white PVC water pipe about 10 inches long which leaves about 6 inches for use as a handle for the man to hold on to and use for precise directional control during use. This handle is critical. The firm core stiffening of the added plastic water pipe gives good control and helps transmit any female response to the man through the dildo. You can actually feel every muscular twitch and contraction of the vagina transmitted through the dildo and the woman can feel any vibrations from an external clitoral vibrator that should be in your other hand transmitted through the dildo. Again, learn to read tiny muscular responses and hip tilting. THE MORE YOU LEARN TO READ HER TINY MOVEMENTS, THE MORE YOU WILL BE ABLE TO DIRECT

TI IE STIMULATION TO THE JUST THE RIGHT PLACE. At first, her reactions will probably not be noticed until you start looking for VERY SUBTLE movements and changes. Again, watch her different vaginal secretions. They tell you the rest of the story. As you become more skillful, you will become more intuitive and be able to interpret more and more subtlety in her movements and sounds. Mark the upper side of the PVC handle with a permanent marker so you know the orientation of the top side when the dildo is buried deep in the vagina. The mark lets you know that the ridge around the head of the dildo is centered at the top which is important to proper female stimulation. It is important to not get any superglue on the surface of the dildo when you install the PVC pipe because the superglue hardens into an abrasive crust in such a way that it ruins the surface for use against delicate vaginal tissue. If you have ever worked with superglue, you know how really runny and messy it is and gets on everything because it squirts very easily in places you don't want it to go if you are not meticulous. It takes only a tiny bit of superglue in just the right places to do the job. We have used the same three most favorite dildos for several years. Buy two, three, or even more. It is fun to have a close duplicate of your own member if you are the typical average of 6 to 7 inches long. Having an extra-large diameter or length or both so your mate can experience that feeling of the legendary "monster" which is also fun and enlightening. Even have at least one which isn't a realistic representation, but instead has some ripples or some other feature that looks interesting to her. Have her involved in the choices. You both will probably end up with a favorite, but will still like to spice things up by changing around for variety. Men are hung up on size, thinking that the bigger, the better, but women can easily be brought to very strong orgasms very effectively with a dildo that is little bigger than a finger. Most women over the long term actually prefer a more normal size used skillfully even though occasionally trying out a bigger size is fun for her even if she probably will be reluctant to admit it. Using one that is near the maximum diameter your mate can comfortably handle is useful for a particular type of stimulating practice, but must be used delicately with plenty lubrication and a gentle touch.

THE A-SPOT TECHNIQUE

Be sure to include a dildo which is typical average diameter, but about 9 inches long for really easy A-spot stimulation pressure at the far upper end of the vagina. During stimulation, her vagina will elongate and what seemed deep to her in the beginning probably is what she will be asking for and she will be asking for firmer pressure at the upper end of her vagina as she becomes more robustly aroused. Just a few deep thrusts at her maximum depth capacity with just the right pressure and timing and will bring her to a rapid and usually an intense orgasm or to a sustained high level plateau just under orgasm that can go on and on. Learn to use your depth of penetration, your timing and pressure skills as you read all of her micro-movements to either make the heightened experience last for her as long as she wants them to last, or use them to finish that particular orgasm when SHE is ready. She will tell you when she is ready in no uncertain terms. Using a dildo in this manner is a delicate skill which actually tugs at the whole clitoral complex and the clitoral root so that it all plays a part in the total stimulus, provides the penetrative rubbing stimulation on the entire G-spot area, stimulates the cervix and aims direct pressure to the A-spot. Add to all of this, a simultaneous gentle direct clitoral head stimulation with your thumbprint or fingerprint, or a vibrator and a powerful and easy orgasm is a sure thing. When you learn to do it right, her orgasms will become much more intense and predictable.

THE G-SPOT AND CERVICAL TECHNIQUE

The G-spot and cervix are in line with each other and whether you are stimulating one or the other depends on the depth into the vagina that you are moving the head of the dildo. Short and slow strokes about an inch or two long in and out as the head of the dildo passes against the #3 G-spot area at the orgasmic rate (.8 Hertz or just barely slower than once per second) will promote a G-spot orgasm. The head of the dildo should penetrate about 2 inches past the pubic bone. A deeper penetration with the dildo pressing against the cervix is accomplished with a deeper stroke of 3 to 4 inches deep at the orgasmic rate so that the dildo head rubs against the hard ring of the cervix. In women who have had children, the uterus is usually dropped and it is important that on the initial insertion, you are very slow and gentle to allow the uterus time to lift up and out of the way before deep penetration. For the umpteenth time, the natural tendency is to try stroking much too fast. Slow down and consciously attempt to hold the rate of .8 Hertz or just barely slower than once per second. It is harder to do than you think because it doesn't feel natural. Be sure to note the necessary angle of the dildo for future reference so you can visualize the same angle of penetration during intercourse. Mix up the depth of penetration of the strokes and make it unpredictable.

The combination of stimulation in all of these areas releases all of the vaginal fluids. Sometimes they are released in a continuous oozing flush and sometimes in a squirting or pulsating flush. When you can consistently do that, you have passed the dildo training and you are ready to see if you can do the same thing during intercourse using Mr. Stiffy. In any case, no matter which way you want to go, you will have a deeply satisfied mate and my guess is that your reward will be quickly forthcoming from a very satisfied and enthusiastic partner for the rest of your life. Give and it will be returned to you!

I will caution you once again, that anything inserted into the vagina should be kept absolutely clean. Dildos should be thoroughly washed with antibacterial soap immediately after every use, rinsed, dried and stored in a clean wrapping such as a clean washcloth or small towel that is changed with a fresh one at each use.

THIS IS EASIER THAN TAXIING AN AIRLPANE

All of these directions sound very mechanical and more complex than it is. It reminds me of the first time I piloted an airplane and was completely intimidated by an instrument panel bewilderingly full of dials and gauges. I didn't understand any of them at the time as I was simultaneously trying to watch all around so the airplane wings weren't hitting anything as I taxied out to the runway. My mind was so overloaded that I couldn't even make the radio call to the control tower at my instructor's command. The instructor had to do it for me because my mind simply couldn't process everything. You will soon be processing it all, and everything will become as natural as breathing.

THE FUN WILL RETURN

You'll catch on soon enough and soon be able to orchestrate it all with precision and confidence. You will no longer need to wear yourself and your mate out by spending long sessions just trying to get something--- anything---to work. You will actually be in control of the situation. Sex will become effortless, easy and fun again. Remember that the dildo training is the training ground for you to use on your intercourse abilities to re-educate your penis to do what it should have been doing all along instead of just poking around wildly and aimlessly in a dark tunnel. You will no longer be just shooting blindly at a target you didn't even know existed. You will be able to mentally picture EXACTLY what is happening inside her as you skillfully ply your new abilities. If she is doing her part to learn how to use her hips and pubic bone and internal muscles, you will both experience the best orgasms you have ever had and that includes those when you were young. That brings us to the next subject.

VAGINAL MUSCLES

There has been considerable attention paid to women's PC muscle (pubococcygeal muscle). It is certainly justifiable because it is important to know about. Training it to be responsive and strong is important. It is the very powerful muscle which is suspended across the pelvis and tightens the vaginal canal by its tension somewhat like a very thick and powerful bowstring attached across the inside of the pelvis. Continence exercises and sex exercises involving the PC muscle are called Kegel exercises. Several devices have been invented for women to strengthen the PC muscle. Some of them are insertion devices of various materials from stainless steel with catch ridges of differing diameters, to flexible and inflatable inserted devices with a gauge for directly reading how strong the contractions are.

THE VAGINAL WEIGHT LIFTERS

One form of exercise is called "vaginal weight lifting". Weights are suspended by a cord from an egg shaped plug which is lubricated and inserted into the vagina and the woman literally squeezes her PC muscle so hard that she can pick up weights with her vagina. Very strong vaginas can lift up to and over 30 pound weights. I would guess that these women are highly prized by their husbands.

Vaginal strengthening is so important to women in some cultures that courses are offered for young women to become so legendarily proficient at vaginal control that they can snag a very rich and powerful husband using their specialized vaginal muscular skills. Russian women go after the new billionaire oligarchs and the high societal levels of some European and Asian countries are noted for using PC muscle skills for social climbing by snagging rich and powerful men. Both partners benefit from vaginal exercise.

Direct stimulation of the clitoral head is the main sexual control switch for the PC muscle during sex, and intermittent clitoral stimulation is one of the best ways to exercise it and make it stronger. The connection is as direct as turning a light switch on and off as you rub the clitoris. Toning it will enhance pleasure for both partners as well as enhance continence if that is an issue. Orgasmic contractions almost always include this muscle as the star performer, but not always. The contraction of the PC muscle constricts the vagina only by squeezing and constricting the distance from the pubic bone to the PC muscle in sort of a pinching action in the front third of the vagina. It does nothing to constrict the vagina by narrowing the sides and does nothing to constrict the upper two thirds of the vagina.

THE VERY VALUABLE VERTICAL VAGINAL MUSCLES

There are two sets of vertical muscles that are independent of the PC muscle that provide the side constriction in the vagina, and I have never seen anything in print that addresses their existence, nor how to awaken them and train them. In almost all women they are dormant and have never been awakened so they simply don't work in most women until they are consciously awakened. Very, very few women even know they have them. They are usually nearly completely atrophied and it takes considerable direct attention to establishing the neural feedback loops to make each of these work. It is sort of like the fact that the little toes on most adults are so atrophied that they can hardly sense them and move them individually sideways. By using direct outward sideways finger pressure on the sides of the vagina just inside the labia minor (inner vaginal lips) and giving the woman something to press against, it will give the first glimmer of their existence. Her first successes will come when she is able to make them twitch. With repeated short sessions, she will be able to control them more and constrict them in twitches until they actually become a regular part of mixed orgasms, giving the male partner a real pleasure with the quick twitches at the outer vaginal opening while the deeper contractions of the PC muscle are also occurring. It is delightful. The deeper and stronger pair of the vertical muscles seem to only be awakened after some experience in all internal vaginal orgasmic combinations and then they become regular and easy. The larger vertical muscles are located just to the front of the PC muscle and are smaller than the PC muscle, but are much larger than the pencil sized vertical muscles located just inside the vaginal opening. They can be trained to be strong and in conjunction with the smaller vertical muscles flexed intermittently with the PC muscles, it all can become a really delightful symphony.

THE NO MUSCLE "RELAXED"ORGASM

I said in the last paragraph that the PC muscle is the star performer in most female orgasms, but not always. As the woman's level of expertise responds to the man's increasing simulative expertise, a second level of orgasms occur more often than not, where orgasms effortlessly just happen without any effort and with a fully relaxed pelvis at the beginning of orgasm. The technique is to purposely NOT flex any pelvic muscles as a pointed exercise. Somehow this also aids in bringing on orgasm. It is almost like a "glowing" stage and it is when the woman is floating along just below orgasm for many seconds to minutes in a near catatonic state. This occurs with either internal vaginal or very gentle digital anal stimulation along with very gentle clitoral head stimulation given simultaneously. It requires a consciously forced relaxed state by the woman as verbally coached by her partner to consciously completely relax her vagina. When it happens it is unmistakable, and you will both definitely know it. These orgasms are very deeply satisfying for both partners. Learning to relax and just let things happen is much more effective than trying to force things to happen by more and more muscle tensing.

James A. Grant

MALE MUSCLES

Men, sorry to tell you, but we are much less physically complex sexual creatures than our wives. Our physical equipment is actually pretty boring in comparison and with our wives equipment and with much less mystery. We are more visually stimulated than they are, so that puts more of our sexual experience in the visual picture projector in our heads. Since our main sex organ is external, it is pretty easy to examine and there is less mystery to it than there is for women's parts.

In men, the penis is attached at its base to our version of a PC muscle. The penis bobs up and down sort of comically when we flex our PC muscle and it makes the whole thing seem a bit difficult to take seriously. Don't blame your mate if it makes her laugh. I think it looks funny, too. That being said, flexing the PC muscle regularly will improve the strength of the bobbing motions of the erection and the erection slightly hardens with PC contractions as these muscles are consciously exercised. Women respond positively to these motions during intercourse and sometimes male PC contractions alone can trigger orgasm for them when you are inside them. When men ejaculate, the PC muscle spasms at .8 Hertz and that motion inside women tends to trigger their orgasm. We respond just the same to their internal muscular movements. One of the biggest points of enjoyment for women according to some surveys, is the internal involuntary flexing of the penis when the man orgasms and the woman experiences that twitching motion of the penis along with the ejaculate being ejected deeply inside them. Men should exercise their PC muscle while sitting. Then practice a few contractions while otherwise motionless inside your partner throughout the session for diversity. That is a good time for her to practice her outer vertical muscle twitching. You both will love it. It is highly erotic to both sexes. In either sex, the stronger and more toned the PC muscle and the vertical muscles in the woman, the better the sex.

CHAPTER IX

ⱺ

PHYSICAL LIMITATIONS

At age 70, most people have some sort of physical limitations which might include among other things, stamina, flexibility, body strength, heart difficulties, joint replacements, or arthritis. My wife and I have had all of those things between the two of us. That might sound pretty decrepit but it is a fact of life as one ages. Our experience is that if you are lucky enough to still be alive at 70, something hurts about all the time and sometimes on any given day it is nice to feel only one form of ache or pain. The trick is deciding what particular pain hurts more on that given day and deal with it by working around it. I know that any young person reading this book will be sure in their mind that it won't happen to them, but I assure you that it will happen to you if you are one of the lucky ones to live that long. When I was young and heard older people say that, I never thought much about it. At 70, it's just part of the day, and it isn't insurmountable, but it is a bit distracting. My wife and I both have the typical mix of infirmities of a 70 year old plus, but there is nothing that is preventing us from experiencing the sex life which is more fulfilling than when we were married at age 18.

You can do the same. Any time your mood is down or you are just having a boring day, I guarantee that having sex will make things brighter, but only after you have learned to be skilled enough to make sex EFFORTLESS AND FUN rather than the ordeal that it might have evolved into over the decades. I like to quote Art Linkletter who repeatedly stated "Old age ain't for sissies." The older I get, the more grateful I become to be allowed to continue experiencing all of the wonderful little things life has to offer us each and every day. The requirement is that we have to be wise enough to recognize the wonderful gift of life and make the most of it every day. We should all be thinking that the best is yet to come. I make it a point to orient my mind to believe that I have yet to experience my best day.

All physical limitations can be accommodated and worked around if both partners are willing. You may have to alter some positions, use plenty of pillows, slow your pace, and above all, LEARN NEW AND MORE EFFECTIVE TECHNIQUES STARTING WITH A "CAN DO" ATTITUDE. TREAT YOUR MATE AS IF THEY ARE THE MOST IMPORTANT THING IN YOUR LIFE BECAUSE THEY ARE!

The length of your remaining years and your vitality demand it. Everyone is capable of having multiple orgasms in the same day or the same session. It is not so much the orgasm itself that is a limiting factor, it is how skilled you become at learning to give and to receive EFFORTLESS ORGASMS without wearing yourself and your partner out by using the wrong attitudes and techniques. The key word here is "EFFORTLESS."

THE YOUNG AND THE EFFORTLESS

This statement is for the younger crowd. The younger you
and your mate put in the effort to learn and practice the skill
of EFFORTLESS ORGASMS by actually learning what the hell
you are doing, the sooner you will both realize that sex is an
absolutely indispensable part of life and you will benefit the rest
of your life with such knowledge. It puts each of you in control
and makes both of you an indispensable and superior sex partner
who is too precious to allow to slip away to someone else. It
makes you both worth more. Think about it. If you learn the
techniques in the previous chapters, you won't need to work at
having orgasms to keep your psyche and hormones balanced,
you will actually find yourself holding back just enough to NOT
have them until just the right moment of your choosing. As you
approach 40 and older, you will begin to see the relevancy of
what I am saying. Make your goal as a young person to become
such a valuable and skilled sex partner that your mate wouldn't
think to leave you. Your replacement would be too hard to find.

BECOME SEXUAL ROYALTY

Imagine how distinctive a woman is that can lift a 20 pound
weight with her vagina and use that to squeeze your penis,
twitch her vertical vaginal muscles, gyrate and scoop her hips,
and shower you with the enthusiasm of a cheerleader. Think of
how sophisticated a man is that knows enough to directly target
and hit every one of a woman's erogenous spots exactly when
and how she needs them to be touched. Sex partners like that
are rare and are just too valuable to not treat like royalty. Once
you attain those skills, the physical demands of sex are easy.

JUST GENTLE EFFORT IS NEEDED TO MAINTAIN SKILLS

My wife and I have had to give up a couple of positions, and sexual practices that we once enjoyed, but we found out that we actually more than replaced them with all new things which we didn't even know existed until recent years. I can't express how much that skills learned in the past 7 or so years have many times more than made up for aging and for the giving up of some of the options of youth.

Light flexibility exercises such as Yoga, Tai Chi or just a light version of the stretching exercises like you did in gym class in middle school go a long way toward keeping you flexible enough to accomplish most sexual positions that are the most effective. Some of you old farts probably remember Jack Lalanne on early morning TV who used a simple chair, a broom, and a couple cans of soup to demonstrate an effective but imaginative regimen of exercise that anyone could do. There are dozens of effective light exercise programs that will keep you fit and flexible. Check out the internet.

Not eating before sex is a help to your full body blood flow since your body isn't shoving the lion's share of your blood to your stomach and intestines to digest your food. The more blood flow to the genitals, the more responsive they are.

My wife and I aren't drinkers, but it is a pretty widely accepted fact that a moderate amount of alcoholic drink can be an enhancement to sex (maybe a single glass of wine). A small amount of alcohol is probably useful in loosening inhibitions. A large amount is not conducive to good sex. I can testify that alcohol is not at all necessary, but if you want to incorporate a bit of it, I see no harm to it.

CHAPTER X

SEX FOR ONE

It is a very sad thing when a person loses their mate and continues to live the balance of their life without the sexual satisfaction their mate provided. Also, a person who has chosen for whatever reason to live life as a single person has special sexual needs. The loss of a mate could have been through death or through divorce, but the sexual implication is the same. All three categories have the choice of having extra marital sex, or the avoidance of complications by handling their sexual needs by themselves through some sort of self-stimulation, or a combination of both. It is a very personal decision, and I understand the gravity and difficulty of the choices. The problem is that our sexual needs continue on for as long as we live. It is imperative that those needs are handled for psychological, mental, and physical health. Self- stimulation may be the best second choice for anyone who is alone sexually. In my opinion, self-stimulation decidedly beats going through life unbalanced mentally and physically and getting conned into a position of vulnerability from people who prey upon your obviously sexually compromised situation for their financial gain. WHETHER YOU THINK SO OR NOT,

THE VULNERABILITY OF A SEXUALLY UNBALANCED PERSON IS GLARINGLY OBVIOUS TO OTHER PEOPLE, ESPECIALLY THE PREDATORS WHO ARE LOOKING FOR THEIR NEXT VICTIM.

We can thank many people in the sex aid businesses for providing many forms and types of devices specifically designed to allow a person (male or female) to handle their sexual needs by themselves. All of these sex devices, or more popularly called "toys" can also be used in all forms of relationships of partners or used for sexual self-satisfaction by one person. As I have previously detailed, they can even be a diversion from sex with your partner for an occasional change of pace and are actually necessary to improve sexual skills. They are available in sex toy shops, from household catalogues, and on the internet. Seeing the array of availability in two or three shops is much more educational than ordering on line because specific differences are much better assessed in person. The people frequenting these shops are just normal people and are not the sleazy types one might expect. Remember, the sex revolution has really changed attitudes to a much more realistic attitude than our generation had grown up with. Various ages and a great variety of people are their customers. All transactions are dealt with in a typical retail setting just like any other store, without immature snickering, and without any judgement. No judgement, no snickering, and no guilt. The people you are likely to see are much more mature about the subject than the rest of us. The following list gives some of the major types and uses of these toys.

DILDOS FOR A SURROGATE

These have already been described and discussed, but just to differentiate them from other devices, I am listing them here again. Any shape or form of a device for insertion into the vagina for stimulation is a dildo. At the crude end of the scale, the device varies from any vegetables which can imaginatively be inserted, to anything remotely cylinder shaped and remotely resembling a penis. One perfume manufacturer saw their sales climb dramatically when they bottled one of their perfumes in a tall bottle with a bulbous end which subliminally resembled a penis. Some dildos are made of clear acrylic plastic, some of clear glass which some women seem to like. Many that are not lifelike penis shapes are mostly shaped imaginatively for specific spots of internal stimulation with gentle curves or ribs. Some of them are clear and allow for the observation of the vaginal interior as the sex fluids start to flow when the various areas inside the vagina trigger their release. At the more sophisticated end, real life castings of erect penises of all shapes, sizes and shades of flesh color made from remarkably lifelike silicone/PVC mixture called cyberskin. They are so convincing that if you close your eyes and feel them, they could be mistaken for the real thing. A few of them are even outfitted to ejaculate a lifelike fluid. Many dildos have a suction cup for temporary attachment to a chair seat or to a wall mirror to provide a stable platform for the woman to move against if she uses them for her self- pleasure and hormone balancing. Many have an internal vibrator which works for some people. It's a good exercise for her to hone her hip movement skills using a dildo with a suction cup stuck to a wall mirror or another slick surface. Fantasy dildos exploit the adventurous fantasies with huge sizes or shapes which some women enjoy. You have to see some of them to believe them. Some of them are very imaginative. The best of cyberskin dildos run less that $100 with the cheaper less realistic ones being $25.

VAGINAS- Anything that the penis can be inserted into, substitutes for a vagina for stimulation and has been used for millennia. The most common thing is the hand wrapped around the penis and moved up and down, usually with some sort of lubrication. Such diverse things as a warmed banana peel, warmed raw meat, silk material, a vacuum cleaner hose, and dozens of other objects have been used.

There are real life castings of various porn stars pelvic areas which are as real as the cyberskin are dildos for women. They have lifelike ortifices molded into them for insertion and typically run from about $100 to $250. Some men use these for self-stimulation and hormone balancing.

An interesting question arises. Is it smarter to control natural biological urges using either of these methods of self-balancing or is it smarter to allow yourself to remain vulnerable to making disastrous financial decisions at a moment of weakness being manipulated by a gold digger that whose real motive is taking advantage of your weakness to get whatever he or she wants (including your money)? Also, is it smarter to risk the possibility of disease by having sex with someone with a history you don't really know?

THE EMBARRASSED PAWNBROKER

A funny true story was of a pawn broker a few years ago who was reputed to have gone to a pawn broker's convention. He got the bright idea while swimming at the hotel pool that he would disconnect the automatic pool cleaner vacuum hose from the hose connector head and stick his penis into the suction end of the pool cleaning system. Bad idea!!! The problem was that the suction was so strong that he couldn't get disconnected and he was "engaged" until help could be summoned to extricate him in the very public forum of the hotel pool. I don't think he was seriously injured, but I would like to have been there to hear him explain his swollen and bruised black and blue penis to his wife when he got back home. A bit embarrassing to say the least.

THE REAL THING IS BEST, BUT

Sex is an activity that is certainly best shared with a loving partner, but there are so many circumstances that life brings that can make that either temporarily or permanently impractical or impossible. In those cases, I believe that we should keep all of the balancing and health benefits in play by regularly stimulating our bodies to keep our hormones in balance. For those of you that would like to question this statement, I will assure you that in private, most men and most women are already doing it. Get over the stigma implanted by twisted and hypocritical dogma and just start enjoying your body as the Creator made you---- without guilt or embarrassment.

VIBRATORS

These range from the simplest battery operated vibrator eggs, a $15 plug in hand held "massager" with various changeable heads from the drugstore aisles of larger stores which are very effective, to more sophisticated and sexually explicit models. The sexually explicit models can be a simple penis shape of all descriptions and might include an internal built in vibrator. We have found that the internal vibrator isn't very effective. Some can have rolling ball bearings for bumpy stimulation, and combination "rabbit" style models which are a combination clitoral stimulation and G-spot stimulating dildo using vibrating appendages resembling little rabbit ears for clitoral stimulation along with the internal vaginal stimulation. Little silicone rabbit ears protrude which are super soft and vigorously vibrate on both sides of the clitoris while the outer layer of ball bearings rotates just under the surface of the shaft along with shaft vibration for G-spot stimulation. Some women really swear by the rabbit ear types and they appear to be very effective for some women. Some women think the vibration inside the vagina using some weak vibrator dildos gets swallowed up and is not effective. I agree. Good vibrators, and vibrator/dildos are inexpensive (+/- $60) and I highly recommend that you try several and experiment with them until you find what works best for you. Be sure you buy the ones that are powerful enough for you. We have found that a cord powered vibrator overall is better because it is always powerful and you never have to deal with a weak battery at just the wrong time when you need it the most.

ANAL TOYS

The gay community was primarily responsible for the development of an array of different shaped anal toys designed to stimulate the prostate in men for strong orgasms and also for prostate milking which is somewhat of a medical procedure as it reduces prostate cancer risk particularly in older men. It also temporarily reduces urinary restriction in some men. They are equally effective for vaginal use and anal use in women. One company makes a high end line of them which are under $100 made of surgical stainless steel. Their weight and heft are part of their appeal for an inertial impact effect bumping against the prostate in men or the G-spot for women. Some toys are in the form of plugs made from various rigid or semi-flexible materials which are shaped to insert an elongated bulb shape past the anal sphincter with lubricant and with a flange to prevent more than a couple inches of entry. The internal sensation is said to give the user a focal sensation which enhances penile stimulation. Sometimes simple dildos are used for the same purpose. If any of this appeals to you, give it a try.

LIFE SIZED SEX DOLLS, ANDROIDS, AND THE NEW FRONTIER OF SEX ROBOTS

There is a serious business emerging in very lifelike full sized cyberskin sex dolls with posable metallic support skeletons so they can be positioned for any desired position. They are complete with pubic hair, lifelike penis or vagina, changeable wigs, choice of glass eyes of different colors and are meant to provide the ultimate huggable and willing male or female sex partner. These run roughly in the $3000 to $6000 price range. I bring this up because coupled with computers already developed by the Japanese and Chinese, our descendants could very likely be looking at these for viable surrogate sex partners. Like I said, it is a brave new world, and if the fixation with social media takes an even bigger bite out of our grandchildren's direct human contacts, it is really not so far a stretch to see that strange reality emerge in a couple of decades. There is currently experimentation with voice interactive technology with artificial intelligence. Kind of creepy!

SYBIAN MACHINES USED FOR HORMONE BALANCING AND SELF-PLEASURE

The extremely effective vibrator/oscillator machine made by the Sybian Corporation is a vinyl covered saddle which covers a strong mechanical movement that provides dildo attachments with a conically rotating motion coupled with an infinitely variable and powerful vibrator. It has several attachments of different penis shapes and sizes and also some dildos which are specifically designed for G-spot stimulation. I could easily see busy professional women who don't want any emotional entanglements, or any other women who want instant stress relief making regular use of these machines. They are very powerful, extremely effective, and pretty loud. They were made famous when Howard Stern, the shock jock radio host had several female models use them to orgasm live on his radio show with all of the verbal sounds of orgasm evident to the radio audience. These machines will produce as many clitoral or G-spot orgasms as the rider can stand. One word of caution---they have a strong enough vibration that I think they should be used with caution and at a very low vibratory power setting by anybody with a hip replacement. These range around $1400 depending on the attachment dildos that are included. The knockoffs are a couple hundred dollars cheaper. They are pretty noisy with a loud buzzing sound at the higher vibratory settings, but they are very effective.

A male counterpart using a vacuum sleeve similar to a cow milking machine is available for men, but I don't have any firsthand knowledge of its effectiveness.

OTHER MECHANICAL MACHINES

There are several thrusting machines that are mechanical using special cyberskin dildos where the length of the thrust and the timing of the thrust is variable and they are used by some women. They are large and cumbersome. One type which is more compact is a thrusting machine made like the Sybian saddle but with a thrusting action rather than vibrating and conical rotating action. I have wondered if the mechanical thrusting action could be a risk if great caution is not also used. These types also seem to be effective for their users, but if I was a woman, I think they would scare me. They are also very large and would be difficult to store discretely.

WATER JETS--- SIMPLE, CLEAN, AND EFFECTIVE

These things can be great if used properly. The most common are some form of hand held shower head sold at the drug store. They usually have several spray settings and even pulsating modes. I'm pretty sure some hand held shower heads were really designed for sex use in mind. Directed on the clitoris at just the right angle, just the right intensity of spray and held just the right distance away with just the right temperature and it is a walking home run. Sex shops have some sprayers with a much wider range of jet spray specifically designed for sexual stimulation and I have found some of them superior to shower heads. They are more effective as sex toys than shower heads are. They are under $30 and worth much more in their effectiveness. Be very cautious because if the spray is too strong, the blood vessels on the delicate tissues particularly around the clitoris head will become engorged and can bleed. The solution is to just use a very delicate tickling spray at the right temperature. It is easy for the pleasant feeling to override the subtle pain from a tiny damaged blood vessel unless someone else is assisting you and watching for it. You may not even know it as it is happening. The vessel damage seems to repair itself, but build up the strength of the jet slowly and don't use it for extended periods in a single session.

CHAPTER XI

KEY IMPORTANT POINTS TO REMEMBER

You have chosen to invest your time into reading this book and I hope you have found some facts you weren't aware of. Now it is up to you to do something positive with those facts. Your need for improvement focus might be in the relationship part of your life, may be in the attitude part of your life, may be in the inhibition baggage part of your life, or may be in the physical skill part of your life. To be sure, all of those categories are important, not only to successfully improve your sex life, but also to improve other areas of your life as well.

Following are some of the key ideas for easy reference.

ATTITUDE

A famous radio announcer, Earl Nightingale, in his highly effective motivational tapes refers to "attitude" as the magic word.

How many negotiations or meetings or conversations are ruined by the wrong attitude being displayed by one of the participants even before he or she first opens their mouth by displaying the wrong body language? The meeting was tainted with the wrong attitude from the beginning and made it impossible for anything constructive to happen. Our attitudes show in our posture, our tone of speech, our facial expressions, and even the way we walk or stand. It is very difficult to hide our real attitudes. We are unconsciously very well adept at sensing body language. Only a positive and open attitude will open doors of conciliation and harmony. Be the one who is the peacemaker by displaying a sincere positive attitude and you will likely be surprised at how your leadership guides any conciliatory improvement.

If the air between you and your mate is clear and you already enjoy a spirit of cooperation, be sure your attitudes are both open to improving your sex skills.

PATIENCE

The longer that an unsatisfactory condition has existed, the longer that it is likely to require consistent effort and patience to correct it. I have purposely written this book in such a way that you are prepared for the difficult challenge you might face in dealing with your mate's reluctance to go on this journey with you. You are both carrying the baggage of decades. We all do. One of you is likely carrying a very heavy load and the other of you doesn't have as much baggage, but you both are carrying emotional baggage. It would include all of the petty insults you have directed toward each other, the insecurities either or both of you have regarding your sexuality, your atrophied or undiscovered sexual tools, your inhibitions, and any negative attitudes you have directed toward yourself, and also would include the sum total of all those same things that you had experienced even before you met each other.

I can't stress how much patience was required for my wife and me to chase and catch the first G-spot orgasm. Even after many decades of what we had both considered good sex, we realized that there was still much room for improvement. After that, things seemed to begin to work progressively easier with a few back steps here and there. Other undiscovered circuits then became evident with considerable experimentation and several other dormant erogenous circuits began to open and become functional. We have since learned something very important. It is the technique of relaxation and a letting things happen rather than trying to make things happen. Eastern religions and disciplines like Tai Chi, yoga, Reiki, and martial arts are based on a simple principle. Sometimes a conscious relaxing of all muscles (pelvic and otherwise) and a "letting go" is the answer when that goal continues to outpace us. LET it happen---don't try to FORCE it to happen. Physical therapists tell us that gains come in tiny increments. That goes for all three parts of our being. There will be plateaus of progress that may last for several weeks and it may appear that there is nothing more to gain. Then something will happen to advance your progress to the next level. Remember your youth when you devoted much time to some pursuit and were willing to accept slow gains as you learned a new sport, a musical instrument, or the study of a completely new subject. The same is true when you are older and it is just as important for you to have that willingness to put in the effort and build your skill slowly. That is the very thing that keeps us young. Keep that spirit of adventure alive by using your patience to accept tiny improvements and the big improvements will follow.

WILLINGNESS TO EXPERIMENT AND TO TALK

Non communication is POISON. That is the beginning of the end whether it is instigated by only one or both partners. The level of communication and the depth of which each partner is willing to divulge the REAL core of any problem or desire will determine the success in eliminating the problem. In other words, each partner must be willing to really bare their soul to the other partner and learn to be totally forthright and honest. Sometimes it is extremely difficult to express the real core of a problem and we settle for dancing around the perimeter of an issue hoping that a solution will magically appear. The tendency is to continue hiding our raw feelings and desires because it is difficult to admit that there is a problem for fear the other person might react badly. It is very difficult for us to expose our personality to a possibility of rejection or ridicule. If open communication is continually rejected, the relationship is already dead. When one partner is brave enough to reach down deeper inside themselves to a more open and truthful level, the odds are that the other partner will tend to follow suit even though it is very awkward and uncomfortable. It doesn't happen all at once. It takes some continued effort and it takes a loving regard for the other person. Novices at discussing sex will be attempting to break through decades of repression and it can be very awkward. Verbally state that it is uncomfortable for you and that you love your partner so much that you are swallowing your pride momentarily for the benefit of the relationship. Any fair minded person will respond positively if YOU are really sincere. PRIDE CAN ALSO BE A KILLER IN A RELATIONSHIP.

Sexual experimentation touches on our most protected thoughts and feelings. All of those long held feelings of inadequacy float to the surface. INHIBITIONS DIE VERY, VERY RELUCTANTLY, and it takes consistent and conscious effort to be willing to recognize them and then to determine to conquer them. As your depth of communication improves with your partner, so will the ease of you each facing your inhibitions. The old Chinese proverb states that "The journey of 1000 miles starts with one step". It is so true of any attempt at self-improvement. I have observed that as people age, they either grow in wisdom and become more at ease with themselves and the world, or the burden of decades of bad decisions and unresolved issues becomes nearly impossible to bear and they become embittered, scowling, and miserable creatures.

In each intimate moment, interject something a little new as your partner opens up to you and then be willing for both of you to bend even though it seems very uncomfortable at first. As you detect your partner exposing something that is obviously difficult to express, it is up to you to carry on to the next step by exposing something equally as difficult as it was for you to tell. You will likely find that exercise is a real turn on as you hear some edgy things from the person you thought you knew like the back of your hand.

EVERYONE has some wild and crazy things that have innocently crossed our minds. THOSE THAT DENY IT ARE LYING. Every person alive has had brief fleeting thoughts of having sex with about every member of the opposite sex and maybe more. There is a sexual component to all human interaction of any kind. Everybody has had them, but nobody talks about them, each of us keeping them in our own heads. We all have kept secret corners of our mind. If we are really honest with ourselves, we all have had thoughts about all kinds of sexually related things but have kept them secret for fear of someone else not accepting them for what they are, fantasy. At what point in our lives do we start facing the real truth and get to know our real truthful selves? Several of the reference books I have read related to sex have had chapters or sections devoted to sexual fantasies and preferences and I came away realizing that my own fantasies and proclivities are somewhere in the center of the bell curve and, all the while, I had thought that mine were pretty outrageous. Turns out that I am actually pretty tame. You will probably find out the same thing about yourself. Once these secrets are verbalized to a partner, they actually lose their sting and their control over us and can become a vital part of the most erotic of our encounters.

One thing that is a distinct advantage when you get older is that you tend to be more truthful with yourself and you have had enough years to examine the veracity of all the dribble that has been mindlessly repeated to you for your whole life. That applies to sex as well as all other things out of the mouths of politicians and other power figures who are after your heart and mind. One of the most useful things I have learned is that there is an agenda behind anyone who is trying to get you to do ANYTHING and it is usually at least a bit more selfish and nefarious than they would like for you to believe. Ask yourself why they are trying to convince you to do anything. When you mature past feeling that sex is bad or nasty you will free yourself from many self-imposed shackles. Through open discussion with your mate you will already be in the self-examination process that leads to the truth.

ENTHUSIASM

Nothing is more infectious than enthusiasm. That is especially true in bed. I don't care what other physical shortcomings we think we have, and we all have them, being an enthusiastic bedpartner fuels the fire like a can of gasoline. Until you are well on your way to improving your technique, a little enthusiasm jump starts the process by letting your mate know that you are ready, willing, and able to do what it takes for better intimacy. It is like a self-fulfilling prophesy. Act like what you want to be and you will soon become what you want to be. Do you remember the coy looks you were capable of when you were young? When was the last time you shot one of those looks at your mate? It is likely that after a couple of those inviting looks, old memories will trigger the imprint of earlier times and your mate will very likely want to jump your bones on the kitchen table. Go with it! An enthusiastic partner is a real turn on and a partner that just lays there expecting all things to happen to them as they lay motionless is boring, spoiled and selfish. All sexual encounters I have witnessed or experienced that are really memorable are with turned on and enthusiastic partners. Your sexuality starts in your brain which releases endorphins that jump start all other sexually related chemicals. THINK SEXY AND YOU WILL BECOME SEXY. You don't become better at something by ignoring it.

REGENERATING OR OPENING DORMANT EROTIC CIRCUITS

On the mental side of things, as I eluded to over and over in previous chapters, discovering and opening dormant erotic circuits is probably the most critical and important thing you can do if your sex life has been anything less than perfect.

The mental baggage we are all carrying from a lifetime of well-intentioned but misplaced indoctrination with its resultant guilt inhibits and limits us. The self-loathing or low self-esteem and self-doubt we have carried with us for a lifetime includes all of the mean or thoughtless words from quasi friends and from enemies. Those thoughtless words have literally shut down some of our confidence and ability to shine at our best. Know thy true self! Re-read this paragraph until it really sinks in and you can have a healthy self-esteem.

All negative experiences are a focal point for a self-image as well as ego and confidence building positive experiences bolster our egos. Negative experiences contribute to shutting down sexual responses. If you haven't been an inward looking sort of person, it is likely that the negatives have accumulated more than the positives, and you may even have some recurring self-doubts about your desirability. The more you can train yourself to look at sex and life in general in a balanced and fair way, the more you will come to that healthy position that "I'm o.k. and you're o.k." and stop being overly critical of yourself and of others.

Once you can be fair with yourself, you can sort through all of the slights and injustices that you have choked down for your whole life and then you can begin building the justified measure of self-love that you deserve. It is then and only then that you will be able to actually reverse some or all of the actual psycho-spiritual and psycho-physical damage that has shut down many of your sexual body reactions and all of your sexual chemicals will be produced, transmitted, received and interpreted by your erogenous zones to allow freedom of sexual expression. NEGATIVE SELF-ESTEEM CHOKES YOUR SEXUALITY. It can result in a total inability to function, the inability to reach orgasm, or dampen the fires of passion in varying degrees which rob you of your full potential harmony and satisfaction. This is one of those things where you'll never fully comprehend what you are missing until you have started to actually make a bit of progress. Your sexual health is part of the result of getting your mind, body, and spirit in balance.

Mature past the foolishness of all of the inaccuracies that you were propagandized with through your life by well-meaning and not so well-meaning power figures. It is understandable that family structures and society as a whole requires limits for young minds, but just as you mature in overall judgement through life, you should shed the inhibitions that no longer serve their purpose. The result is that you will become comfortable in your own skin and become tranquil with the rest of creation. YOU WILL HAVE A SENSE OF SELF-WORTH THAT IS NEITHER OVER INFLATED NOR UNDER INFLATED. Go back to the chapter dealing with establishing the latent erogenous circuits that have always been there, but you didn't know existed until you are CONSCIOUSLY aware of each of them.

SOME MORE INFORMATION THAT IS IMPORTANT TO FULL STIMULATION AND SATISFACTION

So far this chapter has dealt with mental and spiritual factors and they are prerequisites for putting all of the physical techniques into full play. A recap of some of those facts and physical techniques that seriously enhance sexual pleasure are as follows:

SEX IS WET

If that turns you off in any way, get past it. In fact, really good sex is usually very wet and involves the natural secretions of at least 4 female fluids and at least two male fluids. It is easy to wipe off and wash off after you are both satisfied. As you open all of the neural pathways to the female G-spot, the U-spot and the A-spot and become accustomed to the smells of all the pheromones, and hormones, and their associated sex fluids up close, you will automatically begin to react to them as nature intended in the first place. Directly to the point, ONE OF THE PURPOSES OF EROTIC STIMULATION IS TO PROMPT THE BODY TO RELEASE THESE FLUIDS IN PROFUSION. We have somehow come to reject natural secretions as unclean through unfounded religious or societal customs while the rest of the world is bathed in them, each appropriate for its own species for all living things, both plant and animal.

As you become aware of sex fluids, it is perfectly normal to recognize them and allow them to do what they were designed to do in addition to procreation---turn you on and to rebalance your psyche through sexual satisfaction.

When the vaginal wall is stimulated, a milky secretion is released which is the consistency of heavy cream. When the U-spot is stimulated, a super slick nearly clear fluid is secreted which varies from the consistency of honey to the consistency of a very light oil. When the G-spot is stimulated a phenomenon called "squirting" or female ejaculation occurs which is similar to prostate or seminal male fluid. This can be in spurts, or in forceful streams and can be just a few drops or a glassful. It is nearly clear, slightly pearlescent with some particulates in it. When the G-spot is stimulated it makes the woman feel like she has to urinate, but it is really the filling of the Skene's glands with the female prostatic fluid and she will want you to momentarily stop the pressure so she can squirt it out. If your penis is inside her, you will need to pull out for a couple of seconds, and if you are using your fingers, you will need to stop the movement against her G-spot momentarily. When the cervix is stimulated it sometimes secretes a small amount of milky, to ropey, to clearer and slicker fluid that looks similar to the vaginal secretion, but has a slightly different aroma. This may all sound a bit clinical, but these fluids are loaded with all of the things that when released, make a woman return to psychological balance, and if they are not released through sexual stimulation, it can make her a holy terror. Men, we are not much different when our testosterone levels are too high.

NIPPLES AND OTHER VARIOUS PLACES OF INTEREST

When stimulated correctly with just the right touch, most men and women have a strong reaction to stimulation of the nipples. If NOT done at the right time or with the right touch, it can cause a pulling away reaction similar to touching the clitoris immediately after orgasm. A light rubbing, very light twisting or tickling, or sucking invokes a very strong reaction in many people--- both men and women. It sometimes is described as a direct line to the genitals. The nipples are one of the most important things to watch for "micro-movement" signals to tell if the woman is getting on toward orgasm. They will shrivel up and go erect and change continually to reflect the level of stimulation she is feeling. Watch them closely as well as tiny twitches in the inner thighs and twitches of the stomach muscles and internal vaginal muscles. They are collectively the flag that tells you what is happening to her arousal. Some women and some men can orgasm with nipple stimulation alone. I can't overstress how important that nipple stimulation at the right time and with the right technique is to enhance arousal. Use the magic frequency of .8 Hertz for your timing.

Each person has specific fetishes which are peculiar to them and if you don't already know what works for your mate, discuss it and find out. It could be back tickling, foot massage, ear tickling, spanking, hair tickling, kissing (anywhere), armpit tickling, talking seductively, or almost anything you can think of. Each person is different, so just be open minded and accommodate whatever they want.

SLOW BREATHING

Sometimes when things just aren't clicking, you are just trying too hard. Both of you just stop a second and relax and do some slow and conscious deep breathing. It increases the oxygen to your body, brain, and erogenous zones, and it lowers the level of anxiety. ALLOW things to happen in a relaxed fashion. This technique nearly always worked for my wife and me to overcome a preoccupation, or a feeling of just trying too hard. AFTER you have developed some advanced skills, sex will no longer be work. It will be fun again so don't get discouraged. The reward of just one really good G-spot orgasm will recharge you both back to your youth and make you believers. Watching your mate in deep ecstasy is a great reward for the man as well as the woman who is experiencing it and visa-versa. A man will reap many benefits with a sexually fulfilled wife, and a wife will gain many benefits from a sexually fulfilled husband.

PUBIC BONES

The relative position of the pubic bones for both partners is important as a fulcrum so that the man can penetrate the woman at the correct angle to direct the penis to the targeted specific area within the vagina. In the missionary position, if the man's pubic bone is positioned above the woman's, he will rub against more of the U-spot at the top of the vaginal opening and the #1 G-spot area as he thrusts. If the man's pubic bone is lower than the woman's, he will hit the cervix and also the A-spot area if he is long enough to put some pressure against the deepest part of the vagina. Along the way he will hit the #2 and #3 and #4 G-spot area with slightly lowered relative pubic bone position. The angle of penetration is critical to learning advanced sexual techniques. Again, I will stress that it is every bit as much the responsibility of the woman to scoop her hips forward and backward so that her partner is entering her at the correct angle for her effective stimulation. With both partners being aware of exactly what is happening, verbal cuing to each other will make the whole experience effortless and rewarding.

As we age, we tend to put on some pounds and that extra fat layer covers the pubic area and prevents the vigorous firm contact and pressure against the woman's clitoris than is possible with a hard body. This effect can be lessened if the woman holds herself open with her fingers tugging sideways on the outer vaginal lips. The man can also wear a hard rubber ring with little protrusions (sometimes called a French tickler) around the base of his penis which will aid in clitoral stimulation. These are very common and have been around for many decades. Different shapes are available.

WEDGED PILLOWS

Wedged pillows made of firm foam are available for about $20 to $30 on the internet. These alone can alter the usual angle and position of penetration enough to instantly improve your success at stimulating both partners. In the missionary position, the woman places the thick end of the wedge under her buttocks so that it is elevated and cants her hips upward. It is the lazy woman's substitute for learning the skill of hip scooping. They are also very useful to improve oral sex by allowing more varied and comfortable positions for both partners. A little experimentation with these on a rainy day will make both of you forget your troubles and you probably won't even realize that it stopped raining an hour ago.

THE MAGIC OF WATER JETS

The bathtub is a great place for all sorts of sex, especially if you have an extra-large tub that are in many homes today. Although the typical hand held shower jets sold everywhere work, by far the best shower jets are found in sex shops or even on the internet which are specifically designed for sex. They run around $30. They are made to have infinitely variable spray and streams similar to the old fashioned brass twisty garden hose nozzle, but much more gentle. They hook into the same fixture as your shower head or with a common diverter section that hooks between the hand jet and the shower head so you can switch back and forth between the hand jet and the shower head at will. It might require a trip to Home Depot for one of the connector fittings. These things are very valuable to learn about the many different kinds of stimulation. It is really helpful for the man to learn how to use these on his partner. Some really deeply satisfying catatonic eye rolling orgasms by your partner will convince you that they are an important tool in your toolbox. They are invaluable as a training tool for the man to learn about his mate.

CAUTION: Be very cautious to not use too strong or too long of spray on the woman because overdoing it can cause tiny blood vessels to engorge and become sore particularly around the clitoral head and shield. The spray should be continually moved in tiny motions and with a gentle spray and far enough away so that the tissues don't become temporarily inflamed. Don't let this scare you or discourage you, just be vigilant and go gently.

YES, SCOOPING AND HIP ACTION AGAIN ---EXTREMELY IMPORTANT!!

This is so important that if you gained nothing else from this book but this simple technique, you will catapult yourself to nearly the front of the line of desirable sex partners. After carefully studying the sex encounters of many, many couples, THIS ONE THING STANDS OUT AS THE DISTINCTION BETWEEN JUST MARGINAL VERY FORGETTABLE SEX OPPOSED TO SUPERCHARGED AND ALL-ENCOMPASSING SEX. When the woman learns how to rock her hips forward and backward in an enthusiastic scooping action, she controls the contact of her clitoris rubbing on the man's penis and directs the penis to anywhere in her vagina she wants it at her command as the arc of her hips goes back and forward. That is true whether she is on top or on the bottom or even lying on her side. It is highly stimulating to the man and gives her complete control. To the man, it feels like he has tied into a tiger. As she perfects this one motion she makes herself a superior sex partner that drastically elevates her desirability. Nothing will do more for a woman than to learn to use this simple action. I have to impress on you that only a small percentage of women really do this correctly and that is the result of our society's ridiculously prudish attitude so that this information isn't passed on to daughters. All women should be aware of this before their wedding night. THE WORST THING A WOMAN CAN DO IS TO SPREAD HER LEGS AND JUST LAY THERE. That says in a screaming voice "I am sexually ignorant, I am not interested, I am inhibited, I am not interesting, AND I don't really love you enough to try to please you. I can hardly wait until this is over!" I certainly hope that's not the message you want to send.

HOLDING HEELS

Several women use the technique of holding their heels with their hands either on the inside or the outside of the ankles with their legs in the air to raise their pelvis for directional control of the man's penetration to different parts of the vagina. It can be very effective. Try it a few times and see if it is for you and incorporate it as a variant for a little spice. It works easiest for trim women, but is still effective for heavier women.

KNEE PUMPING

Many very effective female sex partners use this technique which is a variation of scooping the hips. In one important way it is different, because it engages the leg muscles and adds inertia to the thrust and hip scoop while focusing some of the neural signals to the erogenous zones. I always think of an upside down bucking bronco ride because it is quite a ride and is always appreciated by the man who definitely will not forget it. In this technique, the woman pumps her knees by folding her legs curled up to her breasts and pumps her knees up and down which effectively pumps her hips in a similar motion to scooping with more inertia. It makes the woman look very involved and enthusiastic and is effective for the mental focus of sensations. It will definitely make you a memorable partner.

THIGH MUSCLE TENSING

The isometric tensing of inner thigh and outer thigh muscles for some reason also seems to concentrate a mental focus on erotic sensations in the genitals for both men and women. It can be done by alternately flexing and relaxing either the inner or outer thigh muscles, or it can be a flexing of either the inner thigh muscles alternating with flexing the outer thigh muscles. You will be surprised at how effective this is when you are stuck at a particular level of stimulation. This can be used hand in hand with deep breathing described above. I don't know exactly why it works, but it does.

ERECTILE DYSFUNCTION DOESN'T MEAN THE END---IT IS JUST THE BEGINNING OF BETTER AND MORE ADVANCED SEX

It can be devastating to the ego of a man that actually considers his hard penis as his symbol of manhood, but sex is just as good for those MEN AND WOMEN that decide to let erectile dysfunction be the beginning to learning some of the other techniques you should have learned when you were young. A man with erectile dysfunction can still orgasm the same as he always could and with just as much pleasure. Go back and re-read the chapter section dealing with the subject. He can give his wife controlled and effortless orgasms by honing his skills with his tongue, his hands, vibrators, waterjets, and with dildos. Any good craftsman has many tools in his toolbox that he uses and several different kinds of tools can accomplish the same goal. The same is true of a man as a sex partner. He has many tools at his disposal, he just needs to bone up (pardon the pun) on how to use them the most effectively. Erectile dysfunction doesn't degrade your sex life in the least UNLESS YOU DECIDE that you will let that happen and you choose to refuse to deal with changing realities. Learning how to give your mate effortless and varied kinds of orgasms that are better than is even possible with a hard penis is a whole new adventure that is as exciting as your first sexual encounters. One study has concluded that erectile dysfunction affects roughly 40% of the men in their forties, 50% of the men in their fifties, and 60% of the men in their sixties and so on until it is almost a certainty in really advanced years. If you live a long life, you will experience it at some time or another. One really disturbing fact is that due to the estrogen mimicking chemicals in computerized cash register receipts and estrogen mimicking plastics additives, even some young men in their twenties are showing signs of diminished sperm count and some beginnings of erectile dysfunction.

A WISH AND A BLESSING

To end this chapter and this book, I wish to say that I hope this book will open the forum of forthright and candid discussion about human sexuality. I wish that it would be the spark that ignites a serious and controlled study by scientists, sexologists, psychologists, sex practitioners, and doctors of all of the things about human sexuality that everyone has seemed to be afraid or embarrassed to openly discuss. May we all learn to discuss sex as a subject worthy of guiltlessly and uninhibited consideration. May we all mature enough and get comfortable enough in our own skins to realize that our Creator meant for us to utilize all the wonderful and miraculous things about our bodies without guilt or shame and celebrate the miracle that sex is that evens us out and helps us cope with life and bond deeply with our mate. It is mankind itself who has warped the Creator's wonderful gift of sex into something that is snickered at as if it was impure. I wish for us to all get over our childish attitudes, immature perceptions, and our inhibitions and treat sex as just another subject much like the discussion of the weather or a discussion of stock market prices.

SELECTED BIBLIOGRAPHY

Blakeway,Jill, LAc Sex Again New York, Workman Publishing 2012

Davis, Michele Weiner, The Sex Starved Marriage. New York, London, Toronto, Sidney Simon and Shuster Paperbacks 2003

Easton, Dossie and Harvey, Janet W. The Ethical Slut (2nd Edition) New York, Celestial Arts, an imprint of the Crown Publishing Group, a division of Random House, Inc.

Foley,Sallie MSW, Kope,Sally, MSW, and Surge,DennisP. Ph.D. Sex Matters for Women, New York, London The Gilford Press 2012

Hite, Shere, The Hite Report, New York Macmillin Publishing Co., Inc. 1976

Kaplan, Helen Singer M.D., Ph.D. The Illustrated Manual of Sex Therapy (Second Edition) Levittown, Pa. Brunner/Mazel 1975, 1987

Kaplan, Helen Singer, M.D., Ph.D. The New Sex Therapy, New

York A Bruner/Mazel Publication in cooperation with Times Books 1974

Keesling, Barbara, Ph.D. Sexual Healing (third edition) Alameda, California. Hunter House Inc. Publishers 1990. Copyright 2006, 1996, 1990

Kinsey, Alfred C., Pomeroy, Wardell B., Martin, Clyde E., Gebhard, Paul H. Sexual Behavior in the Human Female, Volume Two Bronx, New York original copyright 1953 later printed Ishi Press International, Bronx, New York

Kinsey, Alfred C., Pomeroy, Wardell B., Martin, Clyde E., Sexual Behavior of the Human Male (Volume II) Bronx, New York 1948, 2010

Masters, William H., Johnson, Virginia E., Kolodny, Robert C. Masters and Johnson on Sex and Human Loving. Boston, Toronto, Little, Brown, and Company 1982, 1985

Reinisch, June M., Ph.D. The Kinsey Institute New Report on Sex. New York: St. Martin's Press, 1990

Zilbergeld, Bernie Ph.D., The New Male Sexuality. New York, Toronto, London, Sydney, Aukland Bantam Books 1992

Printed in the United States
By Bookmasters